YOGA HAPPY

HANNAH BARRETT

YOGA HAPPY

SIMPLE TOOLS AND PRACTICES FOR EVERYDAY CALM AND STRENGTH

Photography by Cecilia Cristolovean

Illustrations by Eleanor Hardiman

Hardie Grant

QUADRILLE

FOR GILES, JACK AND AMELIE.
YOU FILL MY LIFE WITH LAUGHTER
AND LOVE.

CONTENTS

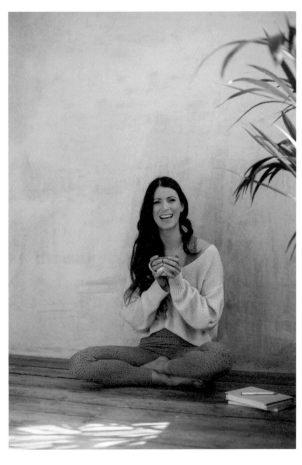
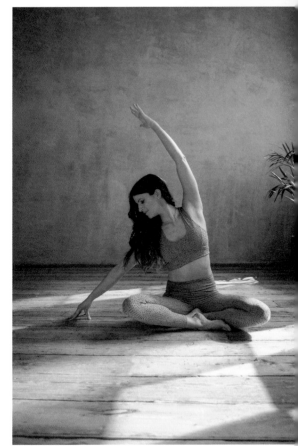
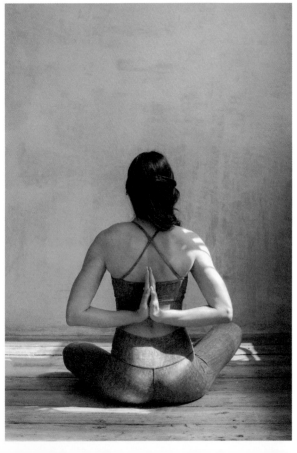
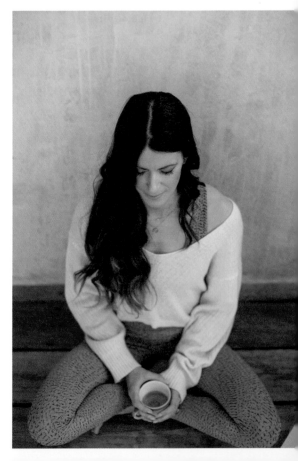

LET'S BEGIN

'YOGA ISN'T SOMETHING WE
JUST DO ON OUR MATS; IT'S
SOMETHING WE LIVE AND BREATHE.
IT IS A WAY OF LIFE.'

HANNAH BARRETT

Ten years ago I never would have believed I'd be sitting here writing a book on how yoga can transform your life and give you the strength and resilience to weather life's fluctuations. I do know, however, that a part of me would have felt very excited because in some way I've always wanted to find the thing in life that would transform me.

I knew exercise was key, I went to the gym religiously and was extremely strong on the outside. But what I lacked was strength on the inside – a sense of knowing who I truly was and trusting that person. I lacked being able to feel extreme comfort in my own company and knowing that when things went as wrong as they possibly could, that I would be okay, that I was mentally strong enough to be okay.

Then, early one morning, something happened that turned my life upside down. When I woke, 35 weeks pregnant, I had no idea that the events over the next few days and weeks would send me spiralling down a path of physical, emotional and mental trauma. That the months ahead would be some of the hardest and darkest I had ever known. But that in the darkness, my life's purpose would emerge and, in time, I would find happiness and contentment like I had never experienced before.

This wasn't the start of my yoga journey. I first started going to yoga classes regularly to help reduce my stress levels before my husband and I started trying for our first baby. At the time I had a demanding job in finance that I loved, but the intensity and long hours were taking their toll and it was clear that stress was getting in the way of what I wanted in many aspects of my life. I had dabbled with the odd yoga class for years with the hope of gaining flexibility (I couldn't even touch my toes at the start), but what I began to learn once I really committed to it, and what drew me in further and further until I became a teacher myself, was that yoga has so much more to offer beyond just the physical.

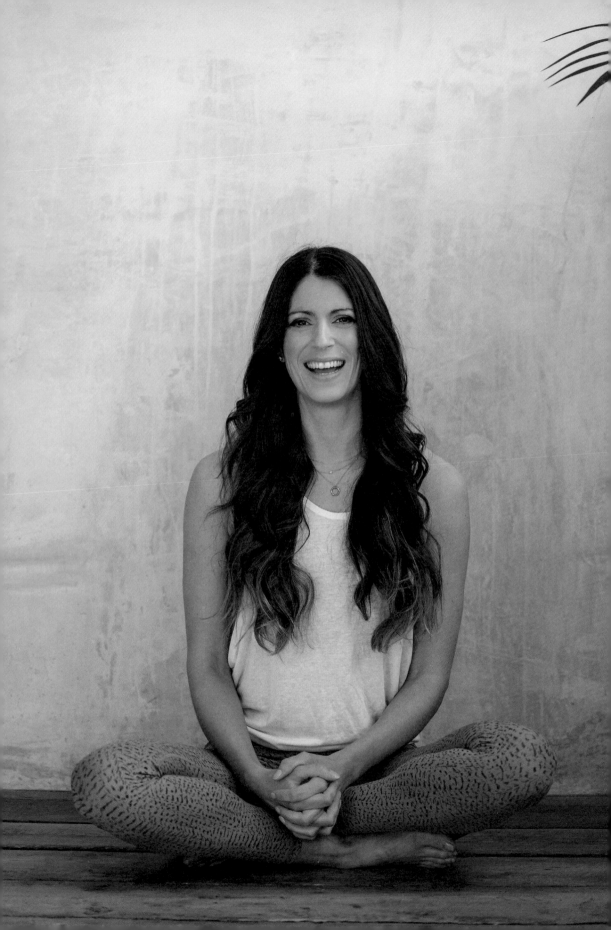

I could push my body through yoga poses on the mat, but it was what stayed with me off the mat – the inner strength, the calm, the clarity – that had the greatest impact. As yoga seeped into my life, I began to absorb the *Yoga Sūtras of Patañjali*, perhaps the most influential yoga book of all time. The word sutra means 'thread' and can be thought of as an observation. Patañjali outlines 196 observations in the *Yoga Sūtras* which are really pieces of wisdom. They put forward yoga's aims, practices, obstacles and the results that can be obtained. In effect, they will help you to live your life with intention, mindfulness and compassion. In the text, he refers to eight 'limbs' of yoga, each of which offers guidance on how to connect mind, body and spirit in order to live with meaning, purpose and freedom.

The physical practice of yoga was designed to facilitate understanding and mastery over the mind. In fact, the only description of the physical postures (asanas) Patañjali gives is *'sthira sukham asanam'* (*sutra* 2.46), meaning that every *asana* should be steady and comfortable. The *sutras* also interpret *asana* as a means to help the body be comfortable sitting in meditation. If we can be steady and comfortable and not distracted by restlessness of the mind or any niggles or pains in the body, we can sit in meditation indefinitely. The combination of the eight limbs of yoga gives us a method to transform how we think, communicate and act by directing our attention inwards, stilling the mind and helping us connect to our true self.

1 **YAMAs** (moral disciplines or restraints)
2 **NIYAMAs** (observances)
3 **ASANA** (physical postures)
4 **PRANAYAMA** (breathing techniques)
5 **PRATYAHARA** (sense withdrawal)
6 **DHARANA** (concentration)
7 **DHYANA** (meditation)
8 **SAMADHI** (enlightenment or bliss)

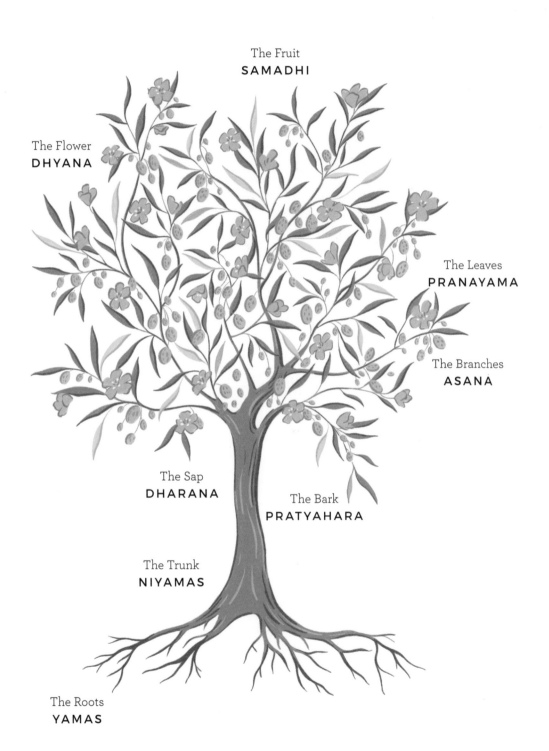

The Fruit
SAMADHI

The Flower
DHYANA

The Leaves
PRANAYAMA

The Branches
ASANA

The Sap
DHARANA

The Bark
PRATYAHARA

The Trunk
NIYAMAS

The Roots
YAMAS

These might seem extremely daunting at first glance but all of the teachings of yoga can be made accessible, not only in the physical practice but for the lessons off the mat too. These ancient concepts can be related to modern life (and over the following chapters I will show you how). Concepts and themes from classes (self-study, truthfulness and non-judgement, to name a few) will follow you after your yoga sessions and over time bring with them inner strength like you've never felt before.

The study of yoga is a lifelong process; even when I started my teacher training, I found myself locked in many negative thoughts. I cared too much about what others thought of me in class, worried they'd think I wasn't 'good' at yoga (in reality other people's attention was purely focused on themselves; they weren't worrying about me). The more I learned in training, the more I learned about myself, and one day I realised my usual thought patterns had changed and I no longer cared what anyone else in class thought about me or my practice. If I wanted to be in child's pose while others were practising handstands, I was fine with that. It was incredibly freeing.

And then my life changed.

It was my second pregnancy and I had gone into it naively thinking it would be a textbook pregnancy like my first. But from about 28 weeks the problems started. Each scan brought with it worrying news and at around 34 weeks we were finally told that my daughter would need to be born early as there was something potentially wrong with my placenta.

When I woke up that night at 35 weeks, I knew something was wrong, but I couldn't put my finger on what it was. Then I began to bleed heavily. I couldn't feel the baby move and I was sure I was going to lose her. I remember shaking uncontrollably for about two hours even after we were told she was doing okay and that it was a suspected partial placental abruption.

After a few days of monitoring it was decided that the risk of a full placental abruption was too high so I was induced. Just over an hour after my waters were broken I was holding my gorgeous and tiny baby in my arms. But things started going downhill very quickly from there.

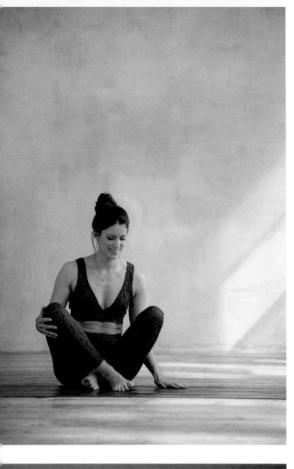

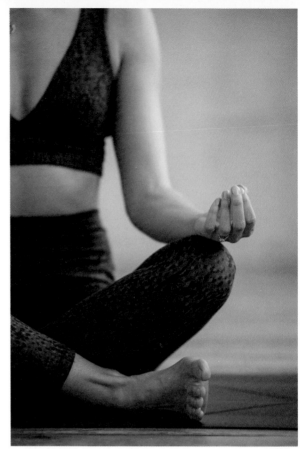

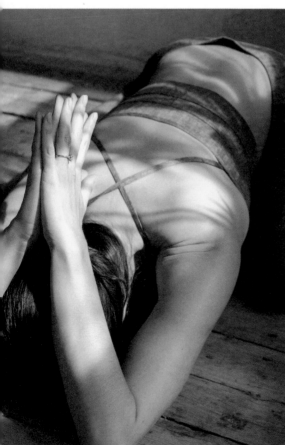

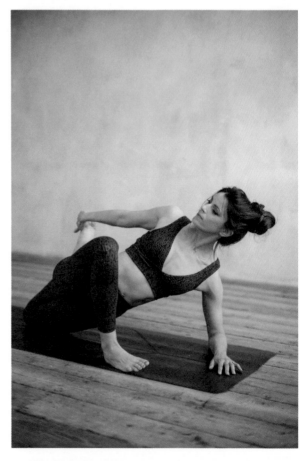

Over the coming days my daughter was to battle sepsis, jaundice, breathing difficulties, eating difficulties and at one stage we were even told there was a possibility of brain damage. It was a living nightmare and I constantly found myself using my yoga techniques for grounding in the present moment because the what-ifs were incomprehensible and the trauma of what happened was too difficult to manage.

The first three weeks of her life, when she was in the neonatal intensive care unit, were terrifying. But we were incredibly lucky and grateful to walk away from the hospital with a tiny but healthy bundle of joy. The fact that my daughter was okay made me bury my trauma even more. It made me think that I didn't have the right not to be okay because I was given the gift of a healthy baby.

Three months later I hit rock bottom and was diagnosed with post-traumatic stress disorder and postnatal depression. And it was in this darkness that step by step I slowly found the light I had always been seeking.

My yoga practice, alongside therapy, helped me recognise myself again, to trust and value myself, and it allowed me to breathe again. I rediscovered who I was, what my passions were and my purpose in life. This started with a mission to help other women through motherhood using the techniques of yoga; to ensure that they didn't experience the sense of being alone that I once had. It then grew to be bigger. This wasn't just about motherhood; it was about *all* humans having struggles that can be eased with yoga. Yoga isn't a magic pill or a quick fix but the tools I share in this book will help you find strength and calm in the chaos of life. Whatever you are struggling with, yoga can help you to build strength to face those battles.

Once I felt reconnected to my body, my mind and most importantly my emotions, yoga started seeping its way into all aspects of my life. My interactions with people and even my inner dialogue became more and more positive. Real growth doesn't happen overnight, but it does come. Yoga has helped literally millions of people to move on from where they are, a little bit at a time. There is no fixed end point – I'm on a constant learning curve and will forever be a student.

Life will *always* be full of incredible highs and the lowest of lows, and as much as I wish I could keep my 'yoga zen' 24/7, I'm also human. I can still lose my cool and feel stressed or inadequate. I'm not immune to emotional trauma and my inner dialogue doesn't always say the nicest things. But what's changed is that I now know what I can do to counterbalance these swings when they happen. Even when I have a dark day, I can see those glimpses of light and I know that I'm going to be ok. Whether I see them through flowing on my mat, taking some time out to breathe or by grounding myself in the present, it doesn't matter. But what I do know is that without returning to these physical and mental practices, the job of healing is more challenging. Yoga is a real lifeline and the resilience it gives me helps me see that it's okay when things are not perfect 100 per cent of the time.

In this book I share the essential toolkit that I *know* works for me and that I've *seen* work for many others who have come to me for guidance. I hope that it provides you with the building blocks for getting in touch with your body and mind, and that it becomes a resource for you to turn to again and again. The beauty of yoga is that it will grow and stretch with you. Best yet, none of what you will find here requires much more space than that which your body already fills. This is the book I wish I'd had in earlier years; I hope it provides you with the resource you need to help you on your own path.

Hannah xx

YOUR YOGA ROUTINE

Here you will learn how to create the perfect yoga routine for your day and what you can expect to find in the rest of this book. I haven't put the stages below in any particular order because you will naturally find the schedule that works for you. I love to start and end my day with meditation and my mindful movement usually happens after the kids are in bed. However, I know lots of people like to move first thing so please play around with the order. You'll learn that yoga is all about tuning in and connecting with what is right for you.

▶ **MOVE WITH INTENTION**
The physical practice of yoga is about mindful movement; learning to work with and understand our limits, maintaining moment-to-moment awareness and recognising where we may need to put in a little more effort or find a little more ease. The first chapter – Move (see pages 19–43) – shares the origins of the physical practice and how to start a consistent and dedicated practice. The following chapter – Let's Flow (see pages 45–63) – offers a collection of sequences to call on depending on your mood.

▶ **FIND TIME TO BREATHE**
The breath is our life force and the essence of yoga. How often do you go about your day paying no attention to your breath? In Come Back to Your Breath on pages 65–77 I outline why connecting with the breath is so important and set out a number of different yogic breathing techniques to create calm, boost energy, promote sleep or find whatever it is you need in that moment.

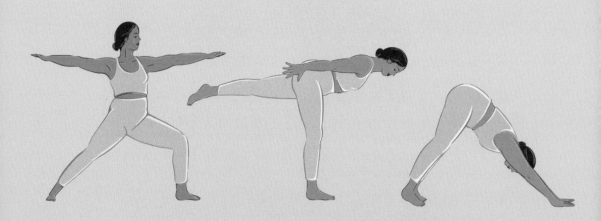

▶ FIND SILENCE

We live in a society of noise and can be constantly on the go, meaning that switching off is extremely difficult. Meditation helps me find calm and has been a saviour in my yoga practice. In Find Silence on pages 79–97 I introduce you to mindfulness and meditation and their benefits and share a number of accessible practices you can incorporate into your daily routine.

▶ JOURNAL

Alongside meditation this is how I start every single day. It doesn't take up much time and it sets the energy and intention for the rest of my day. I talk about gratitude and finding purpose in Self-care and Connection on pages 139–145 and Find Fulfilment and Growth on pages 123–137. Even if you have never journaled before, I challenge you to start now and see the positive impact it has on your life.

▶ SELF-CARE

We often hear that 'you can't pour from an empty cup' and I urge you to believe this is true. The chapter Self-care and Connection on pages 139–145 talks about the importance of a regular self-care routine and how it will positively impact your relationship with others as well as with yourself.

'THE STUDY OF ASANA IS NOT ABOUT MASTERING POSTURE. IT'S ABOUT USING POSTURE TO UNDERSTAND AND TRANSFORM YOURSELF.'

B.K.S. IYENGAR

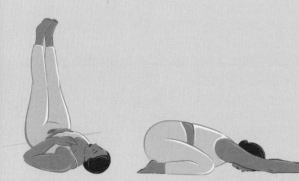

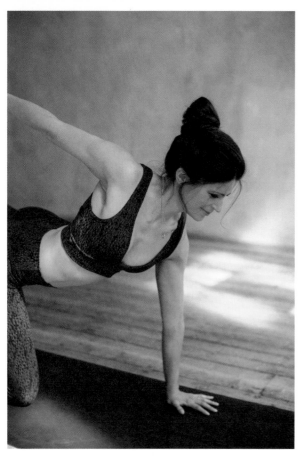

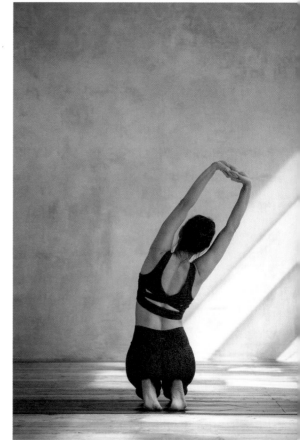

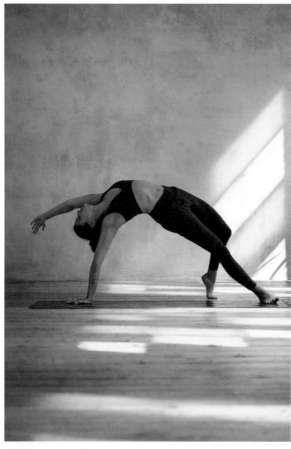

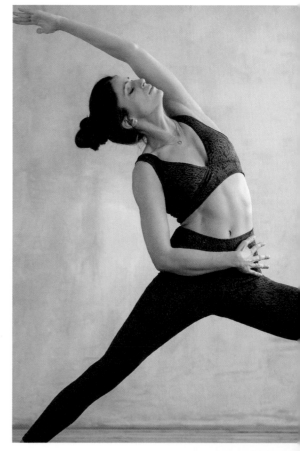

MOVE

'MOVEMENT IS THE SONG
OF THE BODY.'

VANDA SCARAVELLI

I still vividly remember a time when I was unable to touch my toes and holding downward-facing dog pose felt like torture. When I started a regular yoga practice I was strong after years spent in the gym but the movements and postures were foreign and I *struggled*. Part of me wanted to give up and walk away, to return to the gym and the movement patterns I was used to. I am truly thankful that I found the discipline to keep going back to yoga, to keep trying and ultimately fall in love with the practice that would change my life.

Yoga is much more than the postures and physical side. In fact, in Patañjali's *Yoga Sūtras*, the first written text to provide complete guidance on the practice of yoga (see pages 10–11), he mentions *asana* (the physical postures) only three times. They are just one limb of the eight limbs of yoga Patañjali proposes. And what I've found over my years of teaching is that it's often *asana* that draws people in. We start with the body and then begin to access all the other magic that yoga offers.

Yoga starts to change you physically; you become more flexible, more mobile and stronger. Mentally, you gain focus, calm, resilience and inner strength. It starts to seep into your life off the mat and over time you realise that yoga is so much more than just what you do during your practice; you live and breathe it. The yoga postures prepare you for the rest of the practice. They prepare you to grasp the concepts of yoga more easily, but to turn *asana* or postures into yoga you need connection and intention.

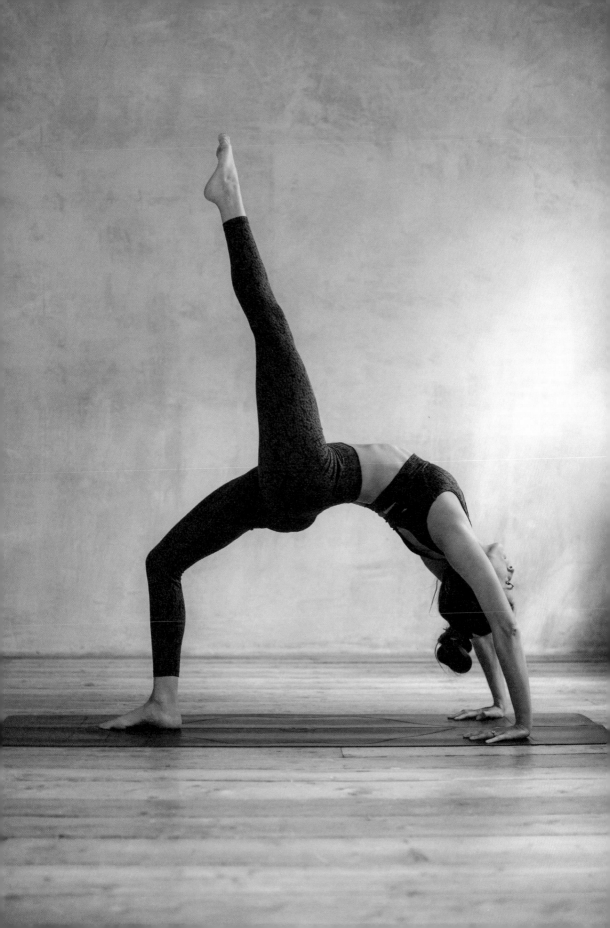

MOVEMENT IS MEDICINE

One of my darkest periods was during and after the premature birth of my daughter. For the first week of her life we didn't know if she was going to make it. When the doctors in the neonatal intensive care unit did their twice-daily rounds, I was asked to leave her bedside so that they could examine her. As you can imagine, this is not what an anxious, traumatised mum wants to do. So, to save my mind from going to wild places, I would get on my yoga mat – my sanctuary, my safe space – and for the three weeks she was in the unit, gentle movement was my medicine.

As my daughter grew stronger and came out the other side, movement continued to be my release. I gave myself a set of go-to yoga flows, breathing techniques and meditations to call on, depending on how I felt. My favourite of these was a restorative sequence of poses I would lie in for five or ten minutes each evening to help open my chest, relieve tension and calm my mind. Even just putting my legs up against a wall for a short period of time, focusing on simply breathing in and breathing out, helped so much.

Yoga *asana* (the physical practice) is something you can truly do anywhere, any time. Five to ten-minute flows are enough to find connection in your mind and body, and ground you in the now. If you've ever tried holding a warrior II pose for a minute or more you will know the connection and resilience you gain; resilience that will stay with you off the mat.

On the following pages, I share tips on starting and maintaining a physical yoga practice and how to overcome some of the common barriers. I'll also give you a whistle-stop tour of the origins of *asana* and what I believe are some of the invisible tools of yoga (the tools you can't actually see but will help you excel at your practice).

In the next chapter – Let's Flow – on pages 45–63 you will find a collection of my favourite short but highly effective flows (yoga sequences) to give you what you need, whether that's a burst of energy, inner strength, restoration, or to relieve some common aches and pains.

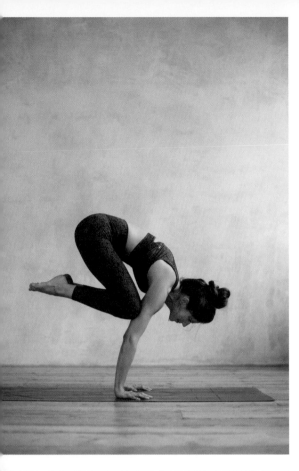

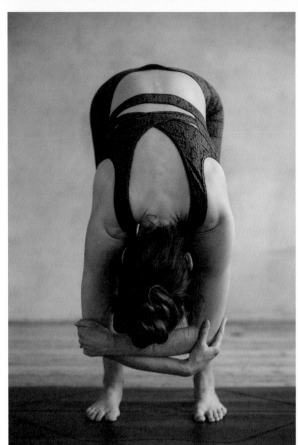

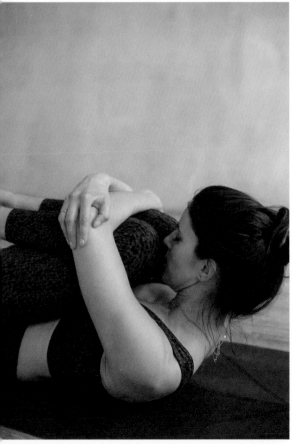

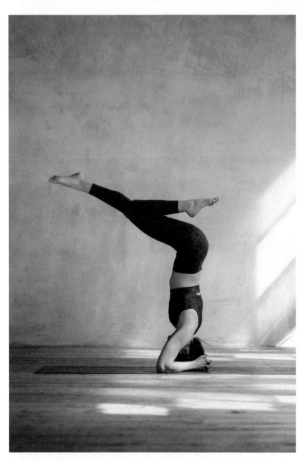

YOGA MYTHS

Believing you need to twist your body into the shape of a pretzel is one of the many yoga myths that have developed over time. I want to air a few of these myths and the reasons people find not to start practising yoga in the hope that if they are on your mind, you can have some comfort that a) you are not alone and b) they should not hold you back from stepping onto the mat or deepening your practice.

▸ YOU NEED TO BE FLEXIBLE

The word yoga means 'to yoke or bind' and is often referred to as 'union'. Yoga is about mindful movement linked to the breath. The physical postures or asanas are designed to purify the body and provide strength, flexibility, mobility and stamina. It's completely okay if you can't touch your toes; you're still performing a forward fold! Flexibility comes over time as a byproduct of yoga, not as a requirement.

▸ IT'S ONLY FOR THE THIN/YOUNG/ETC.

Yoga is for everyone, irrespective of age and body shape. I teach an incredible lady who is 75 and can easily float up into a headstand, and I regularly teach corporate classes where we do the whole flow seated on a chair. Anyone can practise; all you need is dedication and the commitment to keep at it.

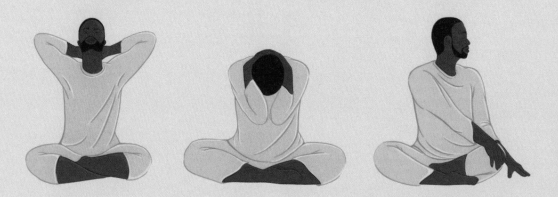

▶ YOGA IS FOR WOMEN

It's true that if you step into a yoga class you may predominantly be surrounded by women. However, traditionally the opposite was true and in India yoga used to be practised almost exclusively by men. It was only when it arrived in the West that it drew a large following among women. Regardless, yoga is all-inclusive and most definitely not gender specific.

▶ YOGA IS TOO EASY/HARD

One of the biggest myths is that every yogi's practice is the same and every yoga class is the same; however there is a huge diversity of teachers and classes. I love how yoga can be made accessible through the use of props and joyous through the use of language. Yoga is even educational, enabling us to learn about the anatomy of the body or the philosophical side to the practice. Every person will be able to find a practice that speaks to them whether that's yin, power or *ashtanga* (the list is endless).

▶ YOU NEED EXPENSIVE TOOLS

There are companies that exist to provide yogis with specialised clothing, mats, props and more. While these can be lovely to have, they are not required. Yoga should be practised in whatever feels comfortable, with space to move, with a mat or without.

▶ IT TAKES TOO MUCH TIME

You don't need to practise for 90 minutes every day to be classified a 'yogi' – I certainly don't. Modern life is busy and it shouldn't be an obstacle to your practice. A five to ten-minute practice is still valuable, will benefit your body and mind and it can make being consistent so much easier.

▶ DOING ADVANCED POSES MEANS YOU'RE BETTER AT YOGA

I used to believe this and when I walked into a yoga class would feel inadequate and inferior to the yogis standing on their hands or sliding into the splits. The poses aren't the goal. Whether or not you can stand on your hands doesn't make you a better or worse yogi than the next person.

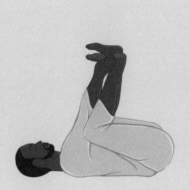
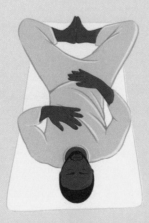
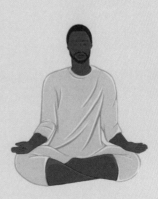

ORIGINS OF ASANA – THE PHYSICAL PRACTICE OF YOGA

The *Yoga Sūtras* is the first written text to provide complete guidance on the practice of yoga. Patañjali didn't invent yoga with the *Yoga Sūtras*; instead it is said that he systemised the ideas and practices already around and compiled them in one place.

As I touched on earlier (see page 10), the *Yoga Sūtras* suggest that *asana* is a means to help the body be comfortable sitting in meditation. When sitting in meditation we strive for stillness, without pain in a relaxed state. But it is surprisingly difficult to sit down for 10 minutes without fidgeting or feeling stiffness or aches. *Asana* is designed to help us purify our bodies and prepare us for meditation and the other limbs of yoga. When we feel suppleness through the body, when the breathing is smooth and the energy flows freely, we can find a relaxed state and start to focus our attention inwards.

JUST START

Starting a yoga practice takes a lot of courage. It is hard, particularly if you're not naturally flexible or coordinated. I urge you to stick with it – over time it becomes easier and you will reap the rewards both on and off the mat. Take photos of yourself practising regularly, particularly of the poses that you find difficult. After a couple of months, when you look back and compare photos, you'll be able to see how far you've come.

If you're reading this thinking, 'I can't touch my toes' or 'I don't look like the stereotypical yogi', know that yoga is for everyone. There is no such thing as a stereotypical yogi and I can honestly say that when I started practising yoga I could not touch my toes. Flexibility, mobility and coordination had never been my friends.

How flexible you are is actually pretty irrelevant. If your hands finally reach the ground in a standing forward fold or your pelvis finally touches the ground in the splits I can promise you that enlightenment doesn't magically happen (although inwardly you will feel the sense of achievement). The yoga poses are not the goal. They are opportunities to look within ourselves – a bit like looking in a mirror – at the way we react, our tendencies and any patterns. Our practice helps us to create space in our mind and body, it helps us find and connect with our true self.

BEGINNERS: WHERE TO START

If you are completely new to yoga, it is extremely beneficial to learn the foundations of the physical practice in a specialised beginners' class setting. This allows a teacher to observe your form, give you guidance and help you understand and discover postures that can at first feel very foreign.

A tip I give every single one of my students is that as you practise, tune in to sensation and listen to how your body is feeling. The point of practising *asana* is not what the pose looks like to someone else watching you; it's the benefit of the pose to *you* and what it does in *your* body.

For example, the aim of a standing forward fold isn't just to get your hands on the floor and your head to your legs. If this does in fact happen but at the same time your back is curled up like an armadillo, you risk injuring your body simply for the glory of getting your hands down. So, when you hinge at the hips, keeping the spine long, the legs and glutes engaged, and you place your hands on blocks or your shins with a bend in the knees, your hands might not be on the floor and your head is nowhere near your legs but this probably feels a whole lot better in your body as well as being a safer way to practise. Over time you'll become more flexible and your hands will get closer to the floor, but that's really not the point. By not cheating and really tuning in, you are laying a foundation for your whole practice.

YAMAS AND NIYAMAS

Learning the principles of yoga will expand and deepen your physical practice in a significant way and they are the key to your success and safety. Two of Patañjali's eight limbs of yoga are the *yamas* (moral disciplines or restraints) and *niyamas* (observances) and they relate to personal obligations to live well, both outwardly in the world and inwardly toward yourself. You may have also seen them referred to as the *yama* and *niyama*; in the West they tend to be referred to colloquially as the *yamas* and *niyamas*. These are the foundations of a yoga practice; imagine them like the roots of a tree. A tree without its roots would not exist.

I give a few examples over the page but in the chapter Find Fulfilment and Growth (see pages 123–137) we will explore lots of ways to apply the *yamas* and *niyamas* both on and off the mat.

'START NOW. START WHERE YOU ARE. START WITH FEAR. START WITH PAIN. START WITH DOUBT. START WITH HANDS SHAKING. START WITH VOICE TREMBLING BUT START. START AND DON'T STOP. START WHERE YOU ARE, WITH WHAT YOU HAVE. JUST... START.'

IJEOMA UMEBINYUO

AHIMSA, OR NON-VIOLENCE, is the first *yama* and a vital foundation for our physical practice. Non-violence doesn't just relate to our actions towards other people, it also relates to how we treat ourselves. Yoga should not be painful. Yes, at times it will be challenging; it may push you in ways you've never been pushed before, but pain is usually your body's way of telling you something is wrong. If your practice is causing pain, then please ease off or stop and speak to a trusted health professional or qualified yoga teacher.

A common injury I have seen over the years is caused by overstretching, which can do lasting damage to our bodies. Flexibility is amazing but with it we need strength. As with everything in life, you want to aim for balance, and we need balance between passive and active flexibility. Passive flexibility is the range of motion in our joints when we use external force, for example, your hands pulling you into a seated forward fold. Active flexibility is the range of motion in our joints with no external force, i.e. mobility.

We want control in our joints. If passive flexibility significantly exceeds active flexibility there is a higher risk of injury, as you won't really be able to control the wide range of motion in your joints. When you are stretching there should be no shooting or sharp pain. You want to feel a stretch in the belly (the thickest part) of the muscle rather than at the attachments (at each end). So I invite you to really tune in to how things feel, paying attention to what feels hard (but in essence good) and what doesn't feel right at all.

SATYA, OR TRUTHFULNESS, is another key to setting a firm foundation in your physical practice. Ask yourself questions such as: are you being truthful in your practice? Are you ignoring an area of your body where you are feeling particularly tight, or an area of pain? Can you find more truth, kindness and compassion towards your body as you move around the yoga mat? Can you tune in and pay attention to what your body really needs?

What you need can change from day to day. Maybe one day you need a powerful flow to burn off energy and to build strength and power, whereas the next day you may need a short restorative flow to calm your nervous system and quiten your thoughts. It sounds simple enough but our mind can take over. It can push us towards the practice it thinks we need, whether that's an obsession to lose weight or gain more strength, or even the opposite. The mind wants to go with the easier option – poses that require the least effort. It's a fine balance that's hard to get right so pay close attention and strive to tune in.

ASTEYA, OR NON-STEALING, invites you to look into whether you are stealing from your physical practice by trying to do more advanced postures before you're ready and have the foundations in place. Can you find patience and enjoy the journey? For example, practising low plank pose (or *chaturanga*) with the knees lifted again and again before you're ready can cause injury in the shoulders. Can you practise patience, drop the knees and build strength and stability though the shoulders as well as find integration in the core before jumping into the full expression of the pose?

SAUCHA, OR CLEANLINESS, can apply on the yoga mat in a number of ways. It includes taking time to focus on alignment, but also being aware of your thoughts as you practise (think of this as internal cleanliness). Are your thoughts negative or destructive? Are they holding you back? For example, 'I'm never going to be able to manage crow pose' may be the thing holding you back from achieving it. I talk more about this on page 133.

APARIGRAHA, OR NON-ATTACHMENT, helps us practise not grasping and can apply to all things – material and within the body. For example, say you're working towards the splits; don't force or push yourself to your limit (notice when the ego tries to take over) and instead stay present in the moment, appreciate where you are now and have faith that you will master the splits when the time is right.

'YOGA IS NOT ABOUT TOUCHING YOUR TOES, IT IS ABOUT WHAT YOU LEARN ON THE WAY DOWN.'

JIGAR GOR

11 TIPS FOR A SUCCESSFUL HOME YOGA PRACTICE

1. **A ROUTINE FOR YOU** Remember that this is your practice. Create the best weekly routine to suit *your* needs and *your* lifestyle.

   Think consistency over quantity. I have found that my students are much more likely to stick to their practice if they commit to say 10 minutes a day rather than trying to squeeze in 60 minutes here and 30 minutes there.

2. **SHORT CAN WORK** Short sessions can make finding the yoga habit a whole lot easier and can still be extremely beneficial and feel amazing.

   When we set ourselves unrealistic goals (for you that could be a 60-minute practice every day) it can lead you to feel like you are failing before you've even started. To avoid discouragement, start small. Form that habit and then see where your yoga journey takes you.

3. **CLEAR DISTRACTIONS** Even if you can only get on your mat for five minutes, try and put your phone away and find a quiet space to take a moment for you.

   As a mum, I appreciate that at times this can be hard, and I spend at least one practice a week with little ones running around my mat (and at times climbing on me!). So, as much as no distractions is amazing, when life gets in the way, embrace it!

4. **GET COMFY** Wear something that doesn't restrict or isn't going to draw your attention away from the practice. Focus is key.

5. **AVOID PRACTISING ON A FULL STOMACH** *Asana* should preferably be practised on an empty stomach. If this is tricky (and for me it often is!) have something light about an hour before you practise.

   In addition, try not to drink water during the practice – it's said that this extinguishes the internal heat we are trying to create.

6. **BREATHE** Try and breathe in and out through the nose as you practise. This may feel strange at first but over time will become easier. Traditionally, *ujjayi* breath is used for *asana* practice – for more on this see pages 32–33.

7. **BALANCE** In *asana* we are striving for the balance between effort and ease (known as *sthira sukha*). This means having a balance of poses that naturally encourage *sthira* or *sukha* – some to build strength and stability and others to create ease.

   We need to find a combination of strength with a suppleness to allow us to bend rather than break. We can also bring this concept into each pose; this is the delicate seesaw between using just enough effort but not so much so that it creates the wrong tension in the body.

   We can also apply the idea to our joints which need to have a balance of strength (*sthira*) and flexibility (*sukha*) around them for optimal mobility.

8. **PAY ATTENTION** Moment-to-moment awareness is key to ensure you get the most benefit from the practice and to ensure it's safe for your body.

9. **RELAX AND UNWIND** Turn your practice into a self-care treat. Put on some of your favourite music, surround yourself with a scent you love and maybe even crank up the mood lighting.

10. **NOTICE WHAT YOU'RE AVOIDING** There's a saying: 'The yoga pose you avoid the most, you need the most.' Notice in your practice what poses you shy away from.

    Ask yourself why and maybe start to include them into your practice more regularly.

11. **THINK LONG-TERM** Practise for the long-term benefits, rather than putting pressure on what you need to achieve right there and then.

    Go into your practice with the view that you want to be doing this when you're 100.

'YOU DON'T PERFORM YOGA. YOU LIVE IT, BREATHE IT, EMBODY IT. WHAT YOGA LOOKS LIKE IS GOING TO BE DIFFERENT FOR EVERY PERSON.'

HANNAH BARRETT

THE INVISIBLE TOOLS

In terms of the physical practice, there are a number of tools that can be extremely powerful but you can't actually see them. They can give you strength, help you find greater connection in your practice and help you balance. Maybe you've heard words like *bandhas, drishti* and *ujjayi* thrown around in classes before but you aren't exactly clear what they mean. I'm going to help you not only understand them but be able to utilise them to help you progress in your practice.

THE BREATH

I go on to talk a lot more about the breath in the Come Back to Your Breath chapter but it can't be ignored in this one as the breath really is fundamental to a yoga practice. Conscious breathing helps to ground us in the present moment and slowing, steadying and deepening the breath helps to reduce stress and increase overall physical and mental health.

As you practise *asana* you want to breathe in and out through the nose. Traditionally a breathing technique called the *ujjayi* breath (also known as 'ocean' or 'victorious' breath) is used and it's an audible breath that's often compared to the sound of the ocean. Whether you're a beginner or an advanced practitioner, the *ujjayi* breath is a powerful technique that can transform your practice. It's designed to lengthen and smooth out the breath for you.

Some yoga teachers will swear by this breath, not allowing you to breathe in any other way. Personally, particularly for beginners, I believe that if it doesn't feel right for you please just breathe in a way that feels comfortable, striving to breathe in and out through the nose as much as possible. I don't generally teach *ujjayi*; I find students often come to it themselves.

With the *ujjayi* breath you inhale and exhale through your nose. The breath requires a slight constriction at the back of the throat (imagine the sound of Darth Vader from *Star Wars*). To help you understand what this is like, the following may be helpful:

▶ Come into a comfortable seated position with a long spine. As you inhale, feel the belly, the rib cage and all the way up to the collar bones expand. As you breathe out, aim to make the exhale a similar length to the inhale.

▶ Take a deep inhale and exhale through the mouth making a quiet, whispered 'hahhhh' sound as if you are steaming up a mirror. This sound requires a partial closure at the back of the throat.

▶ Take another inhale and as you exhale allow the same faint whispering sound of constriction to continue but this time closing your mouth and exhaling through your nose.

▶ Once you have mastered this on the exhale, use the same method for the inhale, gently constricting the back of your throat.

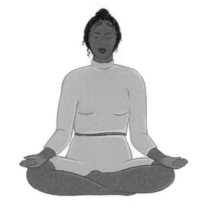

This sound can become a mantra to help you focus your mind. *Ujjayi* will also allow you to notice when too much effort (*sthira*) is being applied and your breathing becomes forced. I find *ujjayi* breathing helps to bring my focus inwards and make my practice feel more meditative.

BANDHAS

If you've been to a yoga class before you may recognise the word 'bandha'. *Bandha* means to lock, bind or tighten. In yoga, there are three *bandhas* commonly referred to and they are thought of as energy locks that direct the flow of energy in the right way.

1. **MULA BANDHA**
   The root lock that stops downward energy escaping from the lower body and redirects it upwards. To activate this lock, lift the pelvic floor (as if you are trying to stop yourself from passing urine or wind).

2. **UDDIYANA BANDHA**
   The abdominal lock that moves energy upwards through the body. To activate *uddiyana bandha*, draw the lower belly up and in.

3. **JALANDHARA BANDHA**
   The throat lock that stops upward moving energy escaping from the upper body. To activate the throat lock, gently nod the chin down and then push the head back in space (like you're trying to give yourself a double chin!).

Jalandhara bandha isn't used in as many postures as *mula* and *uddiyana bandha*. Traditionally it was thought that *mula* and *uddiyana bandha* should be engaged for the whole of a yoga practice. However, doing this can cause overactivation in the deep core, particularly the pelvic floor.

Instead, I teach students to activate these two energy locks on exhales when moving into a dynamic pose or transition that requires more strength in the core (over time it will happen automatically). They shouldn't stay lifted all the time, as the core works in an anticipatory way (anticipating our movements and activating when needed). Particularly in poses of rest and poses that don't need support in the core, I suggest practising letting them go completely. For example, when coming into child's pose, breathe deep into the belly and fully release the pelvic floor.

DRISHTI

Drishti means gaze and is a point of outward focus that helps you bring the focus inwards. Using warrior II as an example; you fix your sight on the front hand as a way of directing your attention to the breath, mind and body. We are so easily distracted by our surroundings, whether it's an area of mess that needs tidying, a clock drawing our mind away or simply a mark on the wall. *Drishti* helps us practise with awareness.

VINYASA

The word *vinyasa* roughly translates as 'to place in a special way'. Many of us have come to see this word to mean the sequence plank, *chaturanga*, upward-facing dog to downward-facing dog, but really *vinyasa* can mean anything. It is the marriage of breath and movement, the linking of one posture to the next.

MUDRAS

The word *mudra* means 'gesture' or 'seal'. *Mudras* are techniques for the flow of *prana* (which means 'life force' or 'vital energy') in the body (see page 70) that can be used in a yoga practice or during meditation. *Mudras* are usually introduced once students have an understanding of *asana*, *pranayama* and *bandhas*. *Prana* is always flowing around and out of our bodies. *Mudras* are thought to direct this dispelled life force back into the body.

STRENGTH IN YOUR FOUNDATIONS

A way to find strength in your yoga practice is to be mindful of your body's foundations, i.e. the parts of the body touching the ground. We want our foundations to be strong and stable to ensure we don't stretch beyond what our body can handle. A couple of pose examples are:

▶ **WARRIOR II** Imagine your feet have four corners and push them into the mat as you lift through the arches of the feet. Notice how energy runs through the legs as you do this, activating the glutes (butt muscles) and igniting the core.

▶ **PLANK** Spread the fingers, grounding through the hands and dialling the hands outwards (like you're screwing jam jar lids in different directions, but your hands aren't actually moving). Feel the strength and stability in your shoulder girdle as you do this.

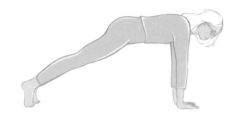

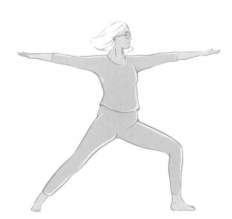

THE SHEATHS
(PANCHA KOSHA)

It is believed that the body is made up of three tiers – the gross body, the subtle body and the casual body. These tiers are then composed of five sheaths or layers (known as *pancha kosha*).

▶ The gross body corresponds to the physical body (i.e. muscles, bones and organs) and the sheath is known as *annamaya kosha*.

▶ The subtle body corresponds to the energetic body and physiological sheath (*pranamaya kosha*), the mental sheath (*manomaya kosha*) and the wisdom body and intellectual sheath (*vijnanamaya kosha*).

▶ The causal body corresponds to the bliss body and spiritual sheath of joy (*anandamaya kosha*).

So how does this apply to *asana*? When we practise *asana* we are striving for integration of all of these sheaths. We want to integrate the body, breath, senses, mind, intelligence and the self with all existence. This isn't something that will come overnight but with faith, and discipline and immersing yourself in all the limbs of yoga it will be achieved.

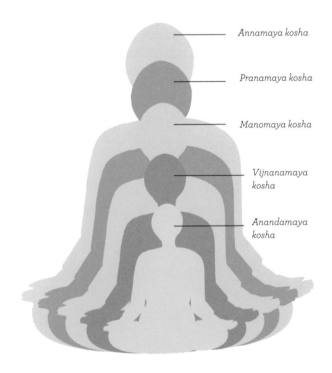

Annamaya kosha

Pranamaya kosha

Manomaya kosha

Vijnanamaya kosha

Anandamaya kosha

NADIS

The word *nadis* comes from the Sanskrit *nad* meaning 'channel' or 'stream'. Just like we have channels for the flow of blood throughout the body, the *nadis* are our channels for the flow of *prana*. According to many Tantric texts, there are thought to be 72,000 *nadis* in the human body, which channel *prana* around the body to every cell. This energy goes to our physical, mental and spiritual development. In essence, the nadis are believed to keep us alive.

Through *asana*, breathing practices and living a yogic life, it is thought that the *nadis* can run clear and free from blockages. Should the *nadis* become blocked or unbalanced, physical, mental and energy issues can manifest. There are three main *nadis*: *sushumna nadi* runs along the spinal column from the base of the spine to the crown of the head; *ida* and *pingala* spiral around the *sushumna* from the base of the spine and end at the left and right nostril respectively.

Sushumna represents consciousness. *Ida* represents the feminine moon energy (cool, intuitive and nurturing) and corresponds to the right-hand side of the brain controlling mental processes. *Pingala* represents the masculine sun energy (warm, rational and dynamic) and corresponds to the left-hand side of the brain controlling vital processes. We all have feminine and masculine energy that runs through us and one way to balance these is through *nadi shodhana* breathing (see page 76).

In Swami Sivananda's book *The Science of Pranayama*, he explains that when the *nadis* are purified there is a 'lightness of the body, brilliancy in complexion, increase of the gastric fire, leanness of the body, and the absence of restlessness'. The unblocking of the *nadis* is a vital function of yoga and leads to optimal health. The practices in this book provide ways to unblock and clear the *nadis*.

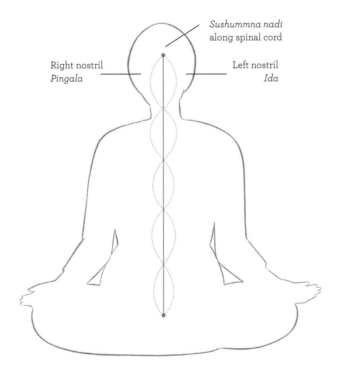

Sushummna nadi
along spinal cord

Right nostril
Pingala

Left nostril
Ida

CHAKRAS

The places where *ida, pingala* and *sushumna nadis* cross correspond to six of the seven main *chakras* in our body (see pages 40–41) with the seventh (*sahasrara*) being just on *sushumna nadi*. *Chakras*, like feelings, aren't physical and can't be held but are visible in our lives through the shape and function of our physical bodies and how we think, feel and react to life both inwardly and outwardly.

The word *chakra* means 'wheel' and can be thought of as a spinning wheel of energy. The seven main *chakras* are thought to correlate with basic states of consciousness. Through habits and external situations a *chakra* can become imbalanced, either deficient or in excess.

With a deficient *chakra*, there's a sense of being physically and emotionally closed off in that area. For example, if *anahata chakra* is deficient it can lead to someone being lonely and withdrawn. When a *chakra* is in excess it can dominate a person's life. For example, if *anahata chakra* is in excess it can lead to poor boundaries and clinginess.

There are many ways to bring your *chakras* back to balance and the physical practice of yoga is one of them. Others include *chakra* meditation, mantra meditation, crystal healing, visualisations and sound healing.

In the brief overview of the *chakras* overleaf I have included some possible mantras to help unblock the relative *chakra*. For more on *chakra* meditation turn to page 96.

Each *chakra* is represented by a colour. Each colour reflects a type of vibration or frequency radiating through the *chakras*. The pathway through the *chakras* is sometimes referred to as the Rainbow Bridge and connects the physical body with the mind and spirit. The *chakras* live in our subtle body (*pranamaya kosha*, see page 36) but can be linked with areas of our physical body too.

If the *chakras* really interest you I highly recommend Anodea Judith's book *Eastern Body, Western Mind*, which delves into the *chakras* and their relation to Western psychologies in great detail.

'THE BODY IS THE VEHICLE, CONSCIOUSNESS THE DRIVER. YOGA IS THE PATH, AND THE CHAKRAS ARE THE MAP.'

ANODEA JUDITH

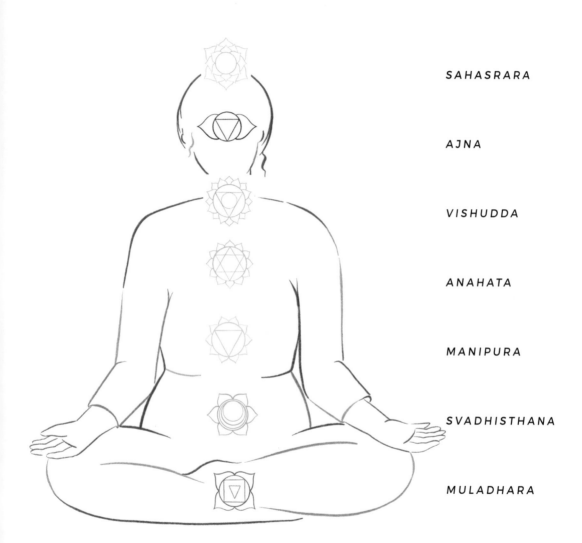

SAHASRARA

AJNA

VISHUDDA

ANAHATA

MANIPURA

SVADHISTHANA

MULADHARA

INTRODUCING THE SEVEN *CHAKRAS*

MULADHARA CHAKRA
Colour: Red
Associated location: Perineum, base
of the spine, at our root
Element: Earth
Function: Survival, security, health, trust,
nourishment and grounding
Mantra/Affirmation: 'I am safe, I am strong,
I am supported'
Action: I am

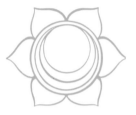

SVADHISTHANA CHAKRA
Colour: Orange
Associated location: Middle of the pelvic bowl
between the pubic bone and coccyx
Element: Water
Function: Our emotional identity, sexual centre
and creativity
Mantra/Affirmation: 'I create my entire reality'
Action: I feel

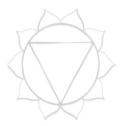

MANIPURA CHAKRA
Colour: Yellow
Associated location: Solar plexus, a couple
of fingers above the belly button
Element: Fire
Function: Our centre of love, compassion
and forgiveness
Mantra/Affirmation: 'I am enough'
Action: I do

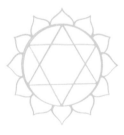

ANAHATA CHAKRA
Colour: Green
Associated location: Heart centre
Element: Air
Function: How we identify with who we
are and what we want
Mantra/Affirmation: 'I am love'
Action: I love

VISHUDDA CHAKRA
Colour: Blue
Associated location: Throat
Element: Ether (or space) and sound
Function: Communication, self-expression and inspiration
Mantra/Affirmation: 'I am open to new ideas'
Action: I speak

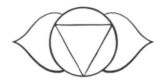

AJNA CHAKRA
Colour: Indigo
Associated location: Third eye
Element: Light
Function: Intuition and imagination
Mantra/Affirmation: 'I trust my intuition'
Action: I see

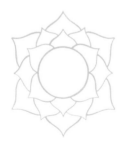

SAHASRARA CHAKRA
Colour: White/ultraviolet
Associated location: Crown of the head
Element: Thought
Function: Energy centre of understanding, universal knowledge and spiritualism
Mantra/Affirmation: 'I am one with the universe'
Action: I know

PROP YOURSELF UP

A prop is simply an object that is used to aid the practice of *asana*. This could be a block to give you more space in half moon pose, a strap to help you get into standing big toe hold, or (my favourite), a bolster to help you melt into restorative postures and let go completely. A mat can even be thought of as a yoga prop.

Yoga props have the capacity to transform your yoga practice. They can also however create a feeling of 'not being good enough' or 'not being flexible enough' and be met with resistance. I can't tell you how many times I have tried to adjust a student in triangle pose by adding a block under the grounded hand to create more space in the body only to walk away and see them go back to grabbing for the big toe.

All bodies are different, we are built differently; our anatomy and our biomechanics are different! So, tune into sensation, notice when you have no space to open the heart and go grab that block. Don't let your ego be the reason you say no to props.

Another way I love to combat the resistance to props is to use them to intensify the practice. Try boat pose sitting on a block or try squeezing a block between the thighs in a sun salutation.

'THE BODY IS THE PROP FOR THE SOUL. SO WHY NOT LET THE BODY BE PROPPED BY A WALL OR A BLOCK?'

B.K.S. IYENGAR

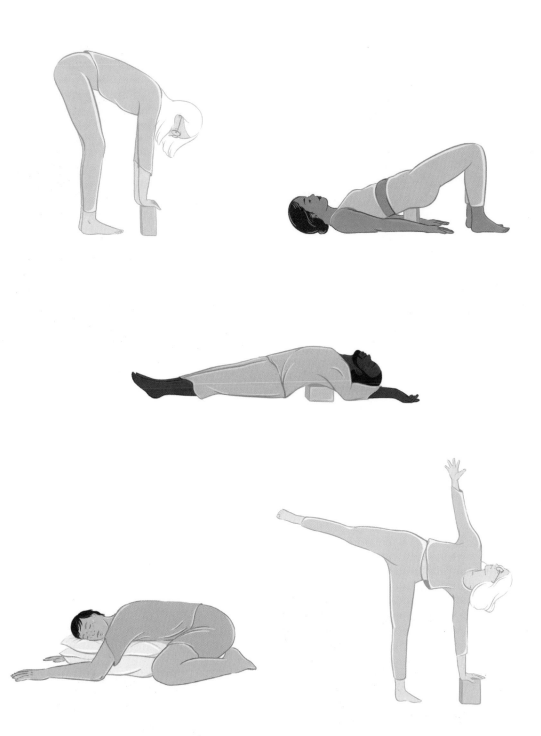

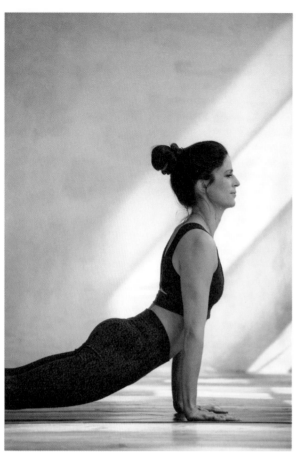

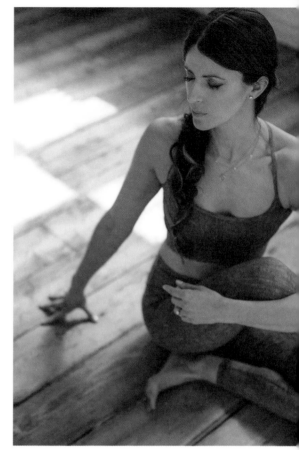

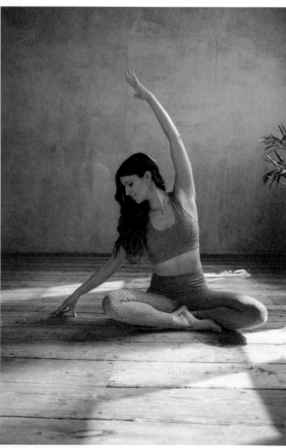

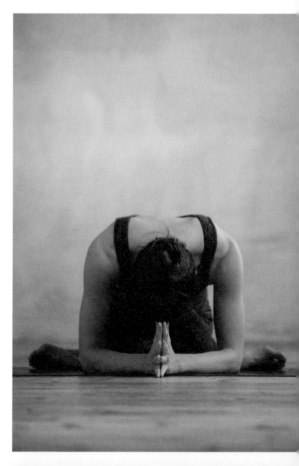

LET'S FLOW

'REMEMBER, IT DOESN'T MATTER HOW
DEEP INTO A POSTURE YOU GO.
WHAT DOES MATTER IS WHO YOU
ARE WHEN YOU GET THERE.'

MAX STORM

Some traditions believe yoga should be practised first thing in the morning before breakfast. In modern times, this doesn't work for everyone and it certainly doesn't work for me. My favourite time of day to practise is 7 p.m. after I have put the children to bed. There's a sense of stillness in the house and my body is yearning to move.

I always take a moment in some kind of restorative pose (usually *savasana*, see page 169) to pause, breathe and to ask myself what it is I *really* need. Most of the time my go-to practice is strength based, but this short pause allows me to check in and be honest with myself. Sometimes it makes me realise that I am running on empty and a more restorative practice is far more appropriate. That quiet moment before I move is in fact the real yoga practice. Sitting, observing, listening. The practice of connection and honesty.

The flows in this chapter are designed to help you whether you want to start your day in the right frame of mind or wind down in the evening. These are my go-to short flows to bring balance to body and mind. We are constantly changing and evolving – what we need one day may be completely different the next (*brahmacharya*, see page 31).

Make these flows your own by modifying them or ramping them up or down depending on *you* and what *you* need. All you have to do is show up on the mat, no more, no less. You will find flows to suit your mood or to overcome negative feelings, to help relieve common health issues, or just to feel stronger.

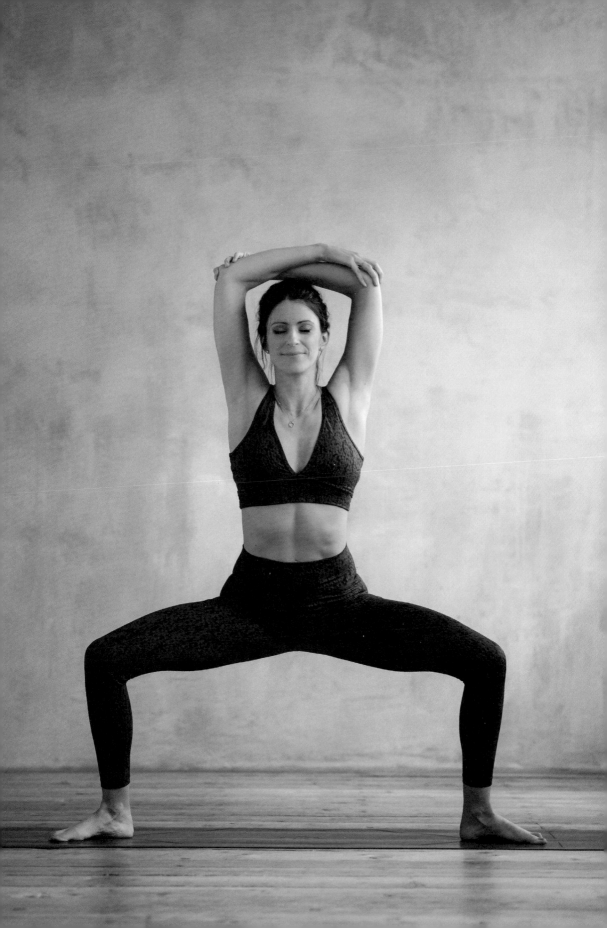

TIPS FOR USING THIS CHAPTER

▶ Turn to pages 152–180 for a detailed appendix breaking down each pose including ways to modify them to suit your body. Yoga should never be painful, so if any of the postures or sequences causes pain then ease off or stop.

▶ For beginners, I highly recommend starting with the energising or calming flow (see pages 50–53 and 54–55). Please be kind to yourself; if you find it too challenging to hold the posture for the designated number of breaths, do as many as you can manage and work up the hold time gradually. This is your body and your practice; take it at the speed and intensity that feels right for you.

▶ I have set out the number of breaths to hold each posture for (although you may need to adjust this to suit you, see above). Keep coming back to the breath as you move between and hold postures, aiming to inhale and exhale to a slow count of four or more. Please don't hold your breath.

▶ On pages 30–31 I set out my 11 tips for a successful home practice. If you haven't read these already, I would highly recommend having a quick look through before you begin.

▶ Those of you who have been to a yoga class might notice that I haven't included the sun salutations (*surya namaskar* A and B) in these flows. The sun salutations set the foundation of *ashtanga* yoga (a style of yoga that was developed by Sri K Pattabhi Jois and T Krishnamacharya in the twentieth century). They are symbolic as well as being rich in physical benefits. If you have more time to spend on your yoga practice they can be a really beneficial addition to the start of a practice, or even a practice in themselves. For details on the sun salutation sequence, I recommend learning them in a class setting.

▶ Try to breathe in and out through the nose in all of these practices (using *ujjayi* breath if you wish – see pages 32–33 for details). If this feels foreign at first, use your mouth to exhale as needed; over time it will become easier.

FLOWS TO TRY

On the pages that follow you'll find five of my favourite go-to flows. Each one is designed to suit what your body may need at a certain time of day or depending on how you're feeling.

ENERGISING FLOW

(pages 50–53)

A 10-15-minute pick-me-up flow for energy and motivation. It's perfect as part of your morning routine to kick-start the day on the right foot. This flow is designed to be suitable for those new to yoga. I introduce you to some of the foundational yoga poses with an invigorating sequence that will build strength, mobility and flexibility.

CALMING FLOW

(pages 54–55)

If you're feeling stressed or anxious, this 10-minute flow will help to balance and connect you to the now. It can also be used to prepare you for a calm and restful night's sleep.

CORE STRENGTH FLOW

(pages 56–59)

A 10-minute fiery yoga flow for when you are short on time but you want to ignite your inner strength and feel powerful.

YOGA FLOW FOR DIGESTION

(pages 60–61)

A flow to help aid digestion and reset your system. This gentle flow will also help create calm and ease in the body.

YOGA FLOW FOR HEADACHES

(pages 62–63)

A short but nourishing flow to bring gentle relief in times when you have a headache.

FREE FLOW

Once you have become more familiar with the postures feel free to create a flow to suit your needs and mood. You can take pieces of the flows above or create something completely different. Self-practice is one of my favourite things, really teaching me to tune in and connect with the body.

ENERGISING FLOW

This is my favourite 10–15-minute flow for when I need energy. It is designed to be accessible to those new to yoga. The sequence introduces you to some of the key yoga postures to help you build strength, mobility and flexibility. Each pose is held for five deep, grounding breaths but if that feels too difficult, feel free to cut the breaths down until you are more familiar with the flow and postures.

WATCH POINTS

▶ Our glutes (gluteal muscles, i.e. butt muscles) love to snooze! From all the time we spend sitting, our glutes are lengthened and not used – which can result in them forgetting to fire or turning off easily. Our glutes are vital for many things, including stabilising our pelvis, so – as strange as it sounds – put your brain in your glutes, which will help build those connections between the muscle and the brain (it's called brain mapping). Common places I see the glutes snoozing in this sequence are warrior II (notice if the front knee collapses in), low lunge (the back glute helps to open the hip), cobra pose, bridge pose and chair pose (make sure the ribs draw in with this last pose as they love to flare).

▶ In bridge pose push down through the feet, lengthen the tailbone and engage the glutes fully ensuring that your pelvis doesn't tip forward, making the lower back overarch. You want to have a neutral spine.

▶ In warrior III the opposite hip to the grounded foot loves to open. Draw the hip down to square the hips. You can place your hands on your hips for useful feedback for this pose.

▶ Plank pose is difficult so please drop the knees if needed; be mindful that your lower back doesn't collapse.

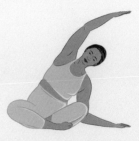

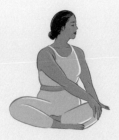

1. SEATED SIDE STRETCHES
Repeat 3 times on both sides.

2. SEATED TWIST
Hold for 3 breaths on each side.

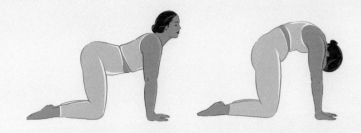

3. CAT/COW
Inhale into cow pose and exhale into
cat pose. Repeat 3 times.

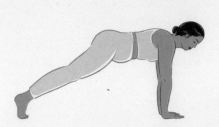

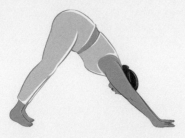

4. PLANK
Inhale into plank and hold
for 5 breaths.

5. DOWNWARD-FACING DOG
Exhale lifting the hips into
downward-facing dog and
hold for 5 breaths.

Continues overleaf ⟫

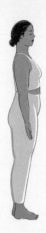

6. MOUNTAIN POSE
Step the feet forward and inhale, lifting into mountain pose for 5 breaths.

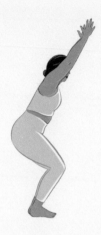

7. CHAIR POSE
Inhale, sweeping into chair pose for 5 breaths.

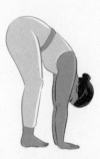

8. FORWARD FOLD
Exhale as you hinge forward into forward fold and hold for 5 breaths.

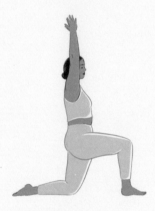

9. LOW LUNGE
Step the left foot back and inhale the arms high into low lunge for 5 breaths.

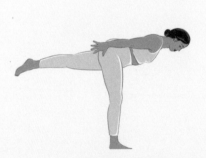

10. WARRIOR III
Lean your weight forward, lifting into warrior III for 5 breaths.

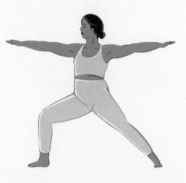

11. WARRIOR II
Exhale as you slowly lower the foot, turning the body to the left side of the mat for warrior II for 5 breaths.

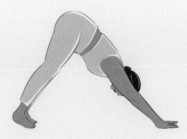

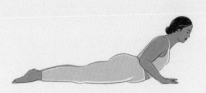

12. DOWNWARD-FACING DOG
Move into downward-facing dog, then step the left foot forward and repeat 9, 10 and 11 on the other side.

13. COBRA
Exhale as you lower onto the belly. Inhale to lift into cobra and hold for 5 breaths.

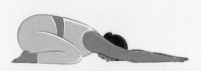

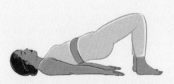

14. CHILD'S POSE
Sit the hips back into child's pose for 3 breaths.

15. BRIDGE
Gently roll on to your back and as you exhale, lift into bridge pose for 5 breaths.

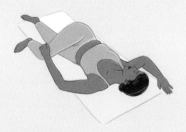

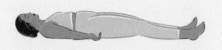

16. SUPINE TWIST
Exhale as you hug the right knee into your chest then slowly lower it to the left side. Hold for 5 breaths and repeat on the other side.

17. SAVASANA
Stay here for 1 minute or more.

CALMING FLOW

If you're feeling stressed or anxious, this 10–15-minute flow will help to balance and calm the nervous system and connect you to the present moment. Take a break away from life and recharge your batteries.

This flow is also perfect to try before bedtime for a restful night's sleep (you can even do the the sequence in your bed). Grab some pillows and prepare to feel relaxed and full of love.

WATCH POINTS:

▶ The first two poses should feel effortless and free. Use as many props as you need to find comfort in each pose so you can focus on the breath and staying present. For example, in reclined butterfly pose, prop up the back and head with pillows and place pillows or blocks under the thighs to reduce pressure on the knees and inner thighs.

▶ Props can also be used in child's pose, placing pillows under the chest can make the pose extremely restorative.

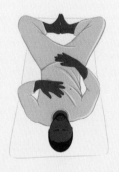

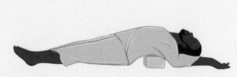

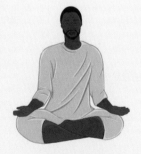

1. RECLINED BUTTERFLY
Release into reclined butterfly pose for 2 minutes, bringing the focus to the breath.

2. RESTORATIVE FISH
Placing a block under the upper back, release into restorative fish pose for 10 slow breaths.

3. SEATED HUMMING BEE BREATH
Gently sit up, cross the legs and take 10 rounds of humming bee breath (see page 77).

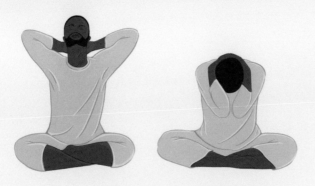

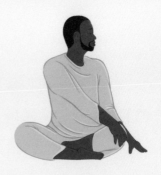

4. SEATED HEART OPENER
Interlace the hands behind the head,
inhale to open the heart, exhale to round
inwards. Repeat 5 times.

5. SEATED TWIST
Hold for 5 breaths on each side.

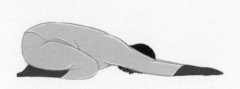

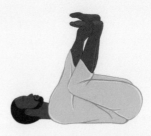

6. CHILD'S POSE
Bring the toes to touch and sit the
hips back into child's pose for
10 breaths.

7. HAPPY BABY
Coming on to your back, take
hold of the feet into happy baby
for 5 breaths.

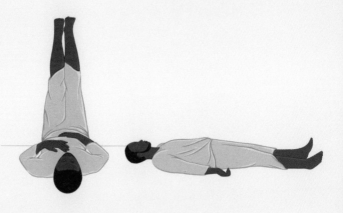

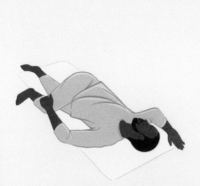

8. SUPINE TWIST
Exhale as you hug the right
knee into your chest, then slowly
lower it to the left side. Hold for 5
breaths. Repeat on the other side.

9. LEGS UP THE WALL *OR SAVASANA*
Chose what your body needs and stay in
the pose for 1–5 minutes or longer.

CORE STRENGTH FLOW

One of my favourite ways to flow, this is a quick and fiery sequence for when you are short on time but you want to feel powerful. Almost every movement we make involves the core, which is why it can cause so many issues when weak or not firing effectively. When activated correctly, it helps to stabilise our spine and support our posture resulting in muscles that can fire more easily and efficiently.

Our core or solar plexus is home to *manipura chakra* (see page 40), the energy centre that represents our personal identity and ego. When *manipura chakra* is in balance we feel energised, confident and powerful.

WATCH POINTS

▶ Connecting to the core isn't simply hugging navel to spine. Think of your core as a unit or web that works together. Part of that unit is your diaphragm (the main breathing muscle) which is why you want to engage the core on an exhale.

To engage the core, on an exhale, lift the pelvic floor (like you're trying to stop yourself passing urine or wind), draw navel to spine, energise the hip bones towards each other and draw the ribs in. As you inhale you don't want the body to be rigid; think about expanding through the belly and ribs, keeping the feeling of strength. As you practise this flow, it will start to happen automatically and you won't have to think about engaging the core.

▶ Although a strong core is beneficial in many ways, we need to practise fully releasing and relaxing the core too. Don't try and do the whole of this flow with the core engaged fully. Be sure to take some deep belly breaths between poses, fully letting go of all engagement.

▶ Boat pose requires a lot of strength – draw the shoulders back, lifting the chest as you find strength in the core and draw the head back in space. If you notice your abdominals doming/bulging or feel like it's too much on the core, either hold the backs of the thighs for support or draw the toes to the floor.

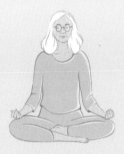

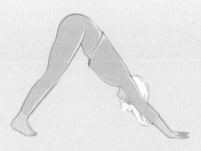

1. SEATED UJJAYI BREATH
In a seated position, take 10
rounds of the *ujjayi* breath
(pages 32–33).

2. DOWNWARD-FACING DOG
Place the hands on the mat
and exhale, lifting the hips into
downward-facing dog.
Hold for 5 breaths.

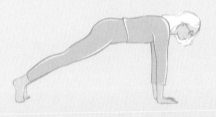

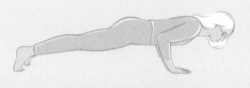

3. PLANK
Inhale into plank and hold for
5 breaths.

4. LOW PLANK
Exhale and lower through
low plank.

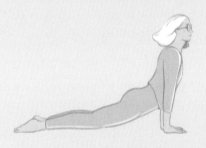

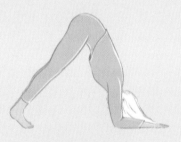

5. UPWARD-FACING DOG
Inhale into upward-facing dog
and hold for 5 breaths.

6. DOLPHIN
Exhale, lifting the hips to the
sky and lowering on to the
forearms to find dolphin pose.
Hold for 3 breaths.

Continues overleaf >>

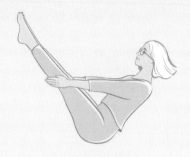

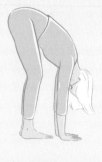

7. BOAT
Come to sit on the mat. Exhale and you lift into boat pose. Hold for 5 breaths.

8. FORWARD FOLD
Bring the feet to the floor and exhale as you lift the hips and fold forwards for 5 breaths.

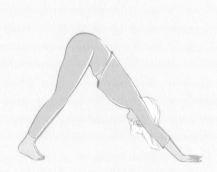

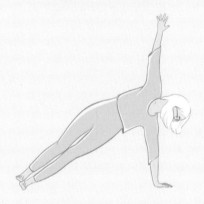

9. DOWNWARD-FACING DOG
Exhale as you step back into downward-facing dog for 5 breaths.

10. SIDE PLANK
Exhale into plank and inhale as you lift the right fingertips to the ceiling, shifting into side plank. Hold for 5 breaths.

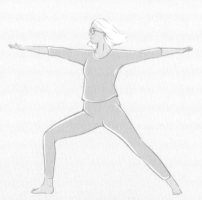

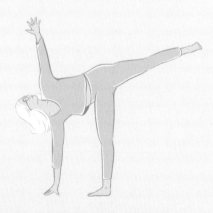

11. WARRIOR II
Exhale as you step the right foot to the front of the mat, lifting into warrior II for 5 breaths.

12. HALF MOON
Inhale, reaching the right fingers forward and down in front of the right foot. Exhale to lift into half moon for 5 breaths.

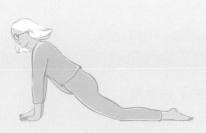

13. LIZARD

Exhale as you lower the left foot
to the ground, bringing the hands
to the inside of the right foot and
lowering the back knee into lizard
for 5 breaths.

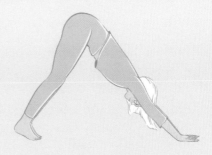

14. DOWNWARD-FACING DOG

Exhale as you step the right foot back
and lift the hips into downward-facing
dog for 5 breaths, then repeat 10, 11, 12
and 13 on the right side.

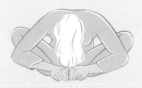

15. BUTTERFLY

Hop forwards and come into a seated
position with the soles of the feet
touching. Exhale as you fold into
butterfly pose for 5 breaths

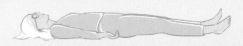

16. *SAVASANA*

Lie back and melt into *savasana*
for 2 minutes or more.

YOGA FLOW FOR DIGESTION

This short yoga flow is designed to aid digestion and reset your system. This sequence will give a gentle massage to your internal organs, create calm and help you keep your lymphatic and digestive system on track. Skip any posture that doesn't feel good for your body.

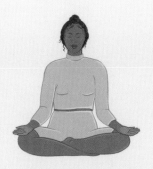

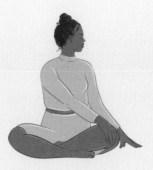

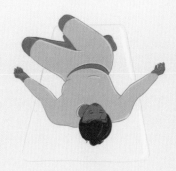

1. SEATED 3-PART BREATH
In a seated position, take
10 rounds of the 3-part breath
(page 75).

2. SEATED TWIST
Hold for 5 breaths on
each side.

3. LAY-DOWN KNEE ROCKS
Coming on to your back, slowly
rock the knees from side
to side 3 times.

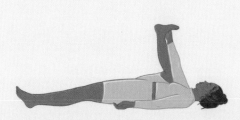

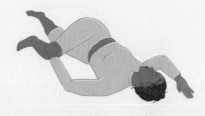

4. HALF HAPPY BABY
Taking hold of the right foot, exhale into
half happy baby and hold for 5 breaths.

5. SUPINE TWIST
Exhale as you hug the right knee into
your chest, then slowly lower it to
the left side. Hold for 5 breaths then
repeat on the left.

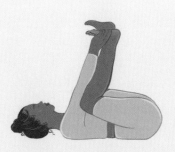

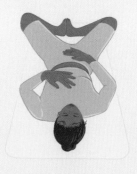

6. HAPPY BABY
Taking hold of both feet,
exhale into happy baby and
hold for 5 breaths.

7. RECLINED BUTTERFLY
Release into reclined butterfly for
10–15 breaths, gently rubbing the
belly in a clockwise direction.

YOGA FLOW FOR HEADACHES

Lots of headaches have a tension and stress-related component so this sequence is all about releasing tension and letting go.

Make sure you're hydrated and only do what feels good for you. These are my go-to poses to bring relief when I have a headache but we are all different. If you're worried about your headache, experience an aura or it continues for an extended period of time, please speak to a medical professional.

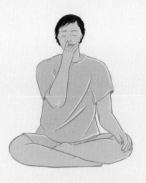 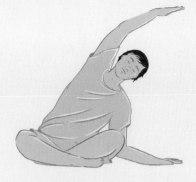 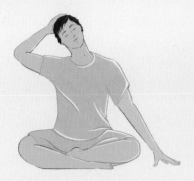

1. SEATED ALTERNATE NOSTRIL BREATHING
In a cross-legged position, take 10 rounds of the alternate nostril breathing (page 76).

2. SEATED SIDE STRETCH
Repeat 3 times on each side.

3. SEATED NECK STRETCH
Taking hold of the head with the right hand, gently exhale into a neck stretch. Hold for 5 breaths, then repeat on the other side.

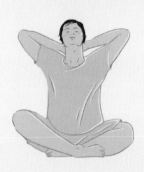 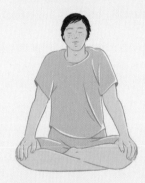

4. SEATED CAT/COW
Interlace the hands behind the head. Inhale to open the heart, exhale to round inwards. Repeat 3 times.

5. SEATED SHOULDER ROLLS
Inhale, rolling the shoulders up towards the ears. Exhale as you release them back and down. Repeat 5 times.

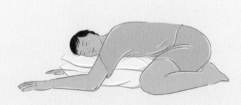 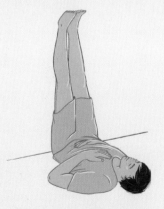

6. SUPPORTED CHILD'S POSE
Bring the toes to touch, place a pillow between the thighs and sit the hips back into child's pose, laying the body over the pillow. Hold for 5 breaths or more.

7. LEGS UP THE WALL
Place the legs up against a wall. With one hand on the heart, one on the belly, take 10–15 breaths or more.

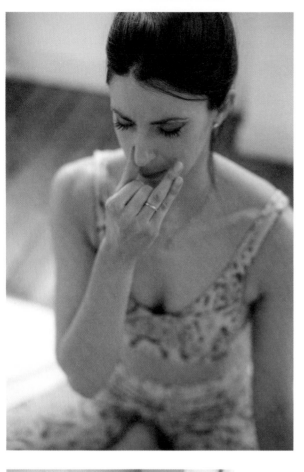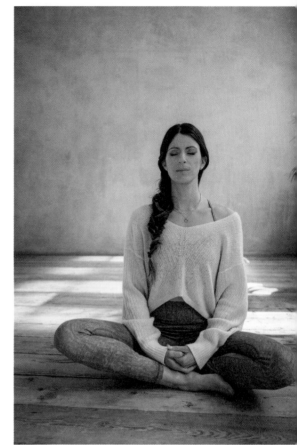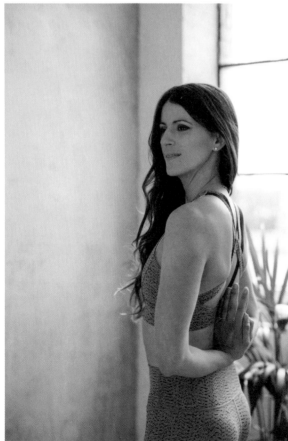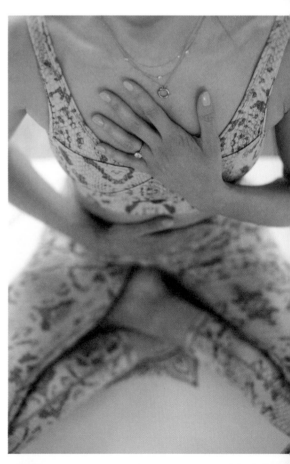

COME BACK
TO YOUR
BREATH

'BREATHE. LET GO. AND REMIND
YOURSELF THAT THIS VERY MOMENT
IS THE ONLY ONE YOU KNOW
YOU HAVE FOR SURE.'

OPRAH WINFREY

One of my favourite things about yoga is simply recognising my breath. Before yoga, I just took breathing to be a basic body function that needed little attention. But I remember once going into a class, feeling overwhelmed and stressed out after a busy day, and the teacher said, 'Stop, slow down and breathe. Focus on the breath going in and coming out.' That simple act completely transformed how I felt – my anxiety started to ease and my mind started to still. I was blown away that we all have this powerful inbuilt tool that we rarely fully take advantage of. So simple but so often forgotten.

We can't survive if we don't breathe. It is both the first and last thing we do on this earth and it is the only system in the human body that we can control both consciously and unconsciously. When I started to pay attention to my breath I realised that my breathing was fast and shallow as a result of the stress I was holding on to in my body. As I explain over the following pages, breathing can work in a circular way – when we are feeling stressed or anxious, for example, our breathing becomes fast and shallow. But we can actually transform how we feel by taking conscious control of our breath; paying attention to slowing and deepening it, feeling the belly, ribs and chest expand with each inhale and a sensation of release on the exhale. This will help you feel calm and relaxed and it is one of the reasons the breath is used as a focus in so many meditations.

If you watch a sleeping baby, see how their lower belly expands as they breathe in and then melts down as they breathe out. We are born with the ability to breathe deeply, fully expanding our lungs, but many of us have lost it, whether it's through the want of a washboard stomach meaning we spend too long rigidly holding in our bellies, or poor posture affecting our ability to take a deep breath.

In this chapter I am going to help you re-connect with your breath and understand how the breath will help you in your life both on and off the yoga mat.

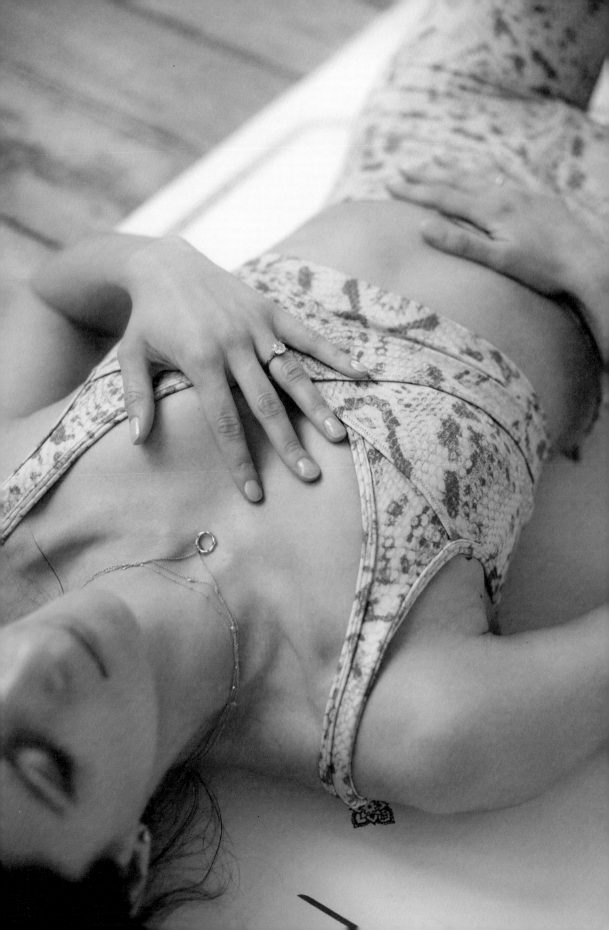

WHY WE NEED TO PAY ATTENTION TO OUR BREATH

You may have heard of the notion that we can live three weeks without food, three days without water, but only three minutes without taking a breath. Our breath is our lifeforce and without it we can't exist. Breathing techniques and paying attention to how we breathe are a way to return balance to the body. Breathing is a key element of health that's often overlooked and can help stop milder issues developing into something more chronic. When you are experiencing stress and anxiety, feel overwhelmed or your mind can't focus, the breath can be an invaluable tool.

Author and alternative medicine advocate Dr Andrew Weil once said, 'If I had to limit my advice on healthier living to just one tip, it would be simply to learn how to breathe correctly.' Although there is a lot of research still to be done and questions to be answered about breathing, the way in which we breathe does matter and there are techniques that can be used as tools for building strength, resilience and to help the body function more optimally.

Breathing is actually the only thing humans can do both consciously and unconsciously. Notice how you can sometimes go for hours (maybe days or weeks even) without paying attention to your breath. Breathing consciously is its own meditation and is the essence of yoga. It helps us to connect with the subtle energy within our body and mind, and grounds us in the present moment. This helps us to let go of the past and/or control of the future and focus just on the 'now', the moment inside the breath.

Take a moment now to be still. Notice what you're feeling in your body and the busy-ness of your mind. Start to breathe with intention, deepening and slowing your breath. Start to settle into stillness and notice where your mind goes. When it starts to wander and leaves the moment, gently notice and bring your attention back to the present using your breath. Observe all sensations. Your breath isn't a simple inhale and exhale – each breath looks different as different parts of your body move as you breathe. Notice the different depths and qualities. Anchor your attention using your breath. Notice how this simple act makes you feel, and how it immediately brings you connection and calm.

When my daughter was a baby, waking three times a night with each feed lasting 1–1.5 hours, initially I would look at my phone, stressing out over lack of sleep and how much time it was taking. I realised I was layering stress upon stress, making it harder to sleep between feeds and I would get up exhausted and the whole cycle would start again. But then I started to practise my breathing in these moments and it not only helped me massively to stop and take stock and hit 'reset', it helped my baby girl calm down too.

What is interesting is that the mind affects the breath but the breath also affects the mind. When the mind is calm, the breath lies steady and peaceful. When the mind is chaotic and moving at 100mph, the breath changes pace, rhythm and depth, often becoming quicker and shallower. This means that we can help to calm the mind by calming our breath.

I try to stop for one to five minutes at least twice a day simply to breathe and 'be'. You can even get apps now that remind you to do this and help you slow and steady your breath. It sounds incredibly simple and perhaps even silly to some, but I challenge you to try it for a few weeks and notice how much you start to look forward to these pauses.

'FEELINGS COME AND GO LIKE CLOUDS IN A WINDY SKY. CONSCIOUS BREATHING IS MY ANCHOR.'

THÍCH NHAT HANH

BREATH WORK

Breath work is conscious control of the breath (rate, rhythm and/or depth) through practices intended to influence your physical, mental or emotional state. Different breathing techniques can therefore be used to help us cope with the different things that life throws at us. We can use our breath as a tool to help calm anger, create energy, reduce anxiety, provide clarity and to help us sleep (see pages 75–77).

As well as the psychological benefits of conscious breathing (creating calm, concentration and presence), changing our breathing pattern can influence physiological factors too. Physiologically, breath work can help to stimulate our parasympathetic nervous system – this is the 'rest and digest system' that allows all parts of the body to relax and recover (the opposite to the sympathetic nervous system, which controls our 'fight or flight' response). So when we are under the influence of our parasympathetic nervous system our breathing is calm, slow and deep. Conversely, when our sympathetic nervous system is taking over, our breath becomes shallow and quickens. But, as I touched on earlier, breathing has a special power over the mind. When we are stressed, we can use the breath as a tool to bring back the calm.

Your breath reflects your emotions, and it can shape them too. Knowing this connection exists allows us to become much closer to controlling our emotional responses – acting rather than reacting – just by changing our breathing. Think back to the last time you received an email or text that made you angry or even upset. How much better is your response when you take a moment to breathe and calm down? It gives you a clarity and a rational mind to respond with.

The beauty of all this is that breathing techniques can be practised anywhere, any time, and at varying levels of intensity.

WHY IS BREATHING SO INTEGRAL TO A YOGA PRACTICE?

Pranayama or breath control is the fourth limb of Patañjali's eight limbs of yoga and it's the heart of our yoga practice. The term comes from Sanskrit, where *prana* means 'life force' or 'energy' and *yama* means 'to extend or draw out'. In *pranayama* therefore, you're using your breath to control the flow of energy and encourage the *prana* into the *nadis* and *chakras* (energy channels and centres, see pages 37 and 38). Just as there are different asanas, there are many different *pranayama* styles that each offer different benefits.

The more *prana* your body has, the more alive it is and if anything blocks this *prana*, it is believed that the body will start to shut down and sickness will follow. There are lots of techniques to unblock *prana* and maintain a steady flow of *prana*, and arguably the most powerful is the breath.

THE BREATH AND YOUR PHYSICAL PRACTICE

Conscious breathing is an integral concept to the practice of *asana*. Without linking conscious breathing and movement, we are not practising yoga, we are just exercising. Keep coming back to the breath as you practise; use it as an anchor to keep you present and in tune with what your body needs; use it to notice when there's too much effort, and not enough ease. As you start to move more dynamically on your yoga mat, can you keep the breath slow and controlled, can you keep it consistent?

As a rule of thumb, try to exhale into postures when you fold forward, or poses that require your core to be strong (like standing forward fold and *chaturanga*). Inhale into back-bending postures where you're opening the chest and expanding the back body (like camel and cobra poses). If you're following a flow like the sun salutations where the movements flow together as one, take more breaths if you need them.

Posture is another area that impacts the breath as it can limit the range of movement of both the diaphragm and rib cage which can result in poor breathing. This means that the breath is going to help in your physical yoga practice but your physical practice will also help improve your posture, which in turn will help your breath!

So how do we breathe on the yoga mat? Funnily enough this can be a fairly contentious topic in the yoga world. Some yogis believe that the only way to breathe as you practise *asana* is to use the *ujjayi* breath (see pages 32–33), however the yoga postures can feel very difficult and foreign for beginners and if you tell them they can only use

ujjayi breath it can be too challenging and even result in them deciding yoga isn't for them. Also, it has been suggested that in certain cases it can overly strain the vocal chords.

Personally, I would recommend that you try to breathe through your nose as you practise. Again, for beginners and people not used to nose breathing, this can be difficult. Don't feel disheartened if you find this hard; instead think of it as a goal to work towards. As long as you continue to consciously breathe and avoid holding your breath, you are practising yoga.

In the *Yoga Sūtras* Patañjali didn't dive deeply into different types of breathing exercises. He instead advises to watch and regulate the breath, 'That [firm posture] being acquired, the movements of inhalation and exhalation should be controlled. This is *pranayama*.' (sutra 2.49).

Once we have mastered the postures, our practice should focus on controlling the inhales and exhales, making them as slow, uninterrupted and smooth as we can. As the breath slows, we can become aware of the energy or *prana*, increase our concentration and gain total awareness of the breath and body.

Although this can be hard, what you will discover is that in time the breath is going to help you advance your practice. It will help to focus the mind, and give you stamina and resilience.

THE SCIENCE

(SIMPLIFIED AND IN A NUTSHELL!)

I think it's helpful to break down a little of the science to show you what is really happening when you breathe so you can see there are actual physical processes at work that you can help control. The power of the breath is truly remarkable!

OXYGEN AND CARBON DIOXIDE

As we breathe in, oxygen enters the lungs and diffuses into the blood and the heart pumps it into our cells. We need this oxygen for everyday functions of the body like moving our muscles and even thinking. When these processes happen, carbon dioxide is produced as a waste product which diffuses into the blood and then into the lungs, and then is expelled from our system as we breathe out.

Deep abdominal breathing encourages full oxygen exchange (i.e. the trade of oxygen for outgoing carbon dioxide) and optimal use of the lungs, meaning our body can function more efficiently. Shallow breathing, on the other hand, means that the lowest portions of the lungs don't get the full share of oxygenated air (which can make you feel short of breath and anxious).

THE MECHANICS

There are two main cavities in our upper body/torso which contain vital organs:

- ▶ **THORACIC CAVITY** The top of the upper body, containing the heart and lungs.
- ▶ **ABDOMINAL CAVITY** Towards the bottom of the upper body, containing the stomach, liver, spleen, kidneys, gall bladder, intestines, bladder and reproductive organs.

Separating both cavities is the diaphragm, a dome-shaped muscle (you can think of it like a parachute). The diaphragm is the principal muscle of breathing. When we inhale, the diaphragm contracts and drops downwards, pressing against the abdominal organs allowing our lungs to expand with air. When we exhale, the diaphragm relaxes and presses back upwards against our lungs, helping them to expel carbon dioxide from our system.

As I mentioned at the start of this chapter, we are born with the knowledge of how to fully engage the diaphragm as we breathe, but life gets in the way. Over time we can end up shifting to chest breathing, leading to less optimal oxygen exchange, and this can result in issues such as higher blood pressure and heart rate.

The good news is that we can strengthen and relearn how to breathe from the diaphragm with a breathing technique called diaphragmatic breathing. As well as increasing oxygen exchange, lowering the heart rate and lowering/

stabilising our blood pressure, it can help promote relaxation and improve the stability of the core muscles (the diaphragm is part of our core!).

To perform basic diaphragmatic breathing:

- Lie on a flat surface with the knees bent and a pillow under the head and knees if required.

- Place one hand on the belly and one on the chest.

- Slowly inhale through the nose, drawing the breath down to the belly feeling it expand under your hands keeping the chest still (the lower ribs will expand laterally).

- Exhale slowly and fully through pursed lips.

- Inhale to fully relax the core and repeat.

Once you have the hang of the technique you can practise this in any position, keeping the shoulders, head and neck relaxed as you do so. Try practising a few times a day for 10 rounds or more.

There are two other diaphragms in the body that are important in yoga – the pelvic diaphragm and the vocal diaphragm. All three diaphragms come together in yoga postures and movements that are coordinated with *ujjayi* breath. *Ujjayi* breath creates a pressure that protects the spine in movements of slow flexion and extension, so coordinating the breath and activation of the *bandhas* creates more stability (*sthira*) in the body as we move around the mat.

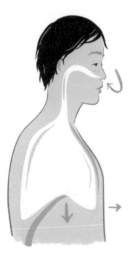

INHALATION

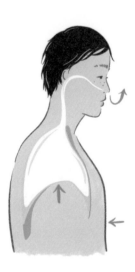

EXHALATION

THE VAGUS NERVE

The vagus nerve is a cranial nerve that runs from the brain through the face and thorax to the abdomen. It's a branching nerve that connects most of the major internal organs between the brain and the colon. It is an essential element of the nervous system, playing a critical role in helping us 'rest and digest'. It's what turns organs on and off in response to stress. When stress levels are low the vagus nerve sends commands to slow the heart rate and breathing, and increase digestion. The reverse is true when stress levels are high. If we can learn how to activate the vagus nerve effectively we can increase vagal tone and become more resilient to stress.

Breathing can help influence the vagus nerve and it's something that we can consciously control. Breathing more slowly will open up communication along the vagus nerve and relax us into a parasympathetic state – one where we are calm, our heart rate is steady and digestion is increased. Interestingly, when I was researching the breath for this book, over and over again I read that there appears to be a breathing 'sweet spot' of an inhale and exhale lasting 5.5 seconds believed to help improve heart rate variability (the steadiness of your heartbeat).

On the flipside, it is also useful to consciously access the sympathetic nervous system (for example by breathing very fast and heavily on purpose) so that we can learn how to effectively turn it off.

BREATHING TECHNIQUES

Below I set out a number of breathing techniques that can be integrated into the start or end of a yoga practice or alternatively can be done as a stand-alone practice when you are in need of their benefits. I also link back to the Let's Flow chapter on pages 45–63 and show you which breathing technique can be a great complement to each flow.

Each of these techniques is a form of *pranayama* to help control the flow of energy/*prana* in the body. As with your *asana* practice, please tune in to how your body feels with these breathing techniques. If you notice any pain, discomfort or unusual symptoms stop and try another technique which is more suited to your body.

For each of these techniques, come into a comfortable seated position with a straight spine and soft shoulders. If you are sitting on the floor, place a cushion or block underneath you if more comfortable. Your eyes can be closed or open, whatever you prefer.

After each session, take a moment to sit with the eyes closed, tuning in and observing how you feel and any sensations.

THREE-PART BREATH

This is my favourite breathing technique and I use it as a tool to find strength daily. The beauty of the three-part breath is that you can do it anywhere – in bed, on the train, walking down the street. I love practising 10 rounds before sun salutations or the Yoga Flow for Digestion (see pages 60–61). Try 5–10 breaths in a comfortable seated position before starting to move.

Suggested benefits include:

▸ reduces anxiety

▸ stimulates endorphins

▸ expands lung capacity

▸ anchors you to the present

▸ helps fight insomnia

Place one hand over the belly and one onto the heart. Take a deep inhale through the nose from the base of your stomach, feeling the stomach expand like you're blowing up a balloon. Keep inhaling, sending the breath upwards through the chest, feeling the ribs moving outwards, sideways and backwards. Finally, send the breath all the way to the collarbones, filling the lungs as full as they will go. Exhale slowly through the nose, feeling the body release all the way down to the base of the stomach.

Aim for each inhale and exhale to be as slow as possible (4–8 counts or longer). Repeat for 10-20 rounds, 2–3 minutes, or for as long as desired.

NADI SHODHANA
(ALTERNATE NOSTRIL BREATHING)

This breathing technique calms the nervous system and brings the right and left hemispheres of the brain into balance. It's a perfect tool to use when you're feeling stressed and seeking stability.

This can be a lovely way to start the Yoga Flow for Headaches (see pages 62–63) to promote balance and calm.

Suggested benefits include:

▸ brings balance to the hemispheres of the brain and energy system

▸ helps correct shallow breathing

▸ relieves stress

▸ brings mental and emotional balance

In a comfortable seated position, tuck the index and middle fingers of your right hand into your palm (*vishnu mudra*) and exhale fully to begin. For some, this can feel uncomfortable – an alternative is to place the index finger and middle finger between the eyebrows (to the third eye; see page 41 for more on this).

Bring the right thumb to your face and close the right nostril. Take a full and slow inhale through the left nostril. Close the left nostril with the ring finger then release the right nostril and exhale slowly and fully. Take a full and slow inhale through the right nostril. Close the right nostril with the thumb then release the left nostril and exhale slowly and fully. This is one cycle.

Repeat for 8–10 cycles trying to even the breath, aiming for an equal length of inhale and exhale. After your practice ends, bring the breath back to a natural rhythm and take a moment to tune in and notice how you're feeling and any sensations arising.

Traditionally *nadi shodhana* also includes breath retention. For those new to the *pranayama*, it's best to focus only on extending the inhales and exhales and aiming for an equal ratio as set out above. Retention is best learned with the guidance of a teacher.

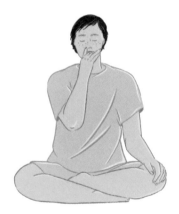

UJJAYI BREATH
(OCEAN BREATH)

On pages 32–33 I set out brief details on the *ujjayi* breath breathing technique, also known as the 'ocean' or 'victorious' breath. This breath is a heating breath helping you warm up the body. It also helps you find balance between strength and calmness and is commonly used whilst practising *asana*.

This breathing technique can be used for all the flows on pages 50–63. It can also be effective as a stand-alone practice if you're in need of an energy boost, and to focus the mind. Come into a comfortable seated position and try 10–12 rounds to relieve tension and anchor you into the present moment.

Suggested benefits include:

▸ the heat created in the body from *ujjayi* breath is said to help detoxify the body and relieve tension

▸ calms and quietens the mind

▸ anchors you to the present moment

▸ increases energy

For details on how to perform this breathing technique, see pages 32–33.

BHRAMARI
(HUMMING BEE BREATH)

Bhramari is a large black Indian bee. This breathing technique is known as the 'humming bee breath' due to the humming sound made on the exhale. It can be a powerful tool to help relieve frustration, anxiety and anger. Personally I also find this breath really useful to quieten the mind. When I have a hundred thoughts running through my head and need to create pretty much instant focus I use this breath as a tool to drown out the mental chatter and go within.

Bhramari can be helpful in times of insomnia so this technique is a great start to the Calming Flow (see pages 54–55). Try 5–10 rounds in a seated or lying down position before starting the flow.

Suggested benefits include:

▸ relieves stress

▸ calms anger and frustration

▸ strengthens the vocal chords and throat muscles

▸ can help insomnia

For the basic form of *bhramari*, sit in a comfortable seated position and take a few breaths, tuning in and observing the body and mind. Inhale slowly through the nose to prepare and release the exhale as a medium to low, slow hum in the throat, like the murmuring of bees, extending the breath for as long as possible. Notice the sensation of the vibrations on your throat, mouth and teeth. Tune in fully to the breath. Try repeating for 6–10 breaths.

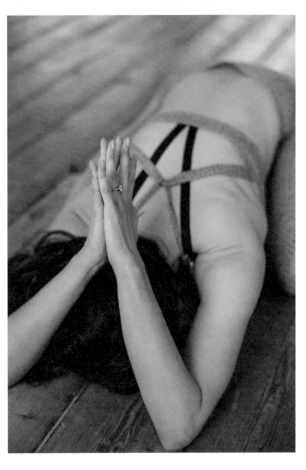

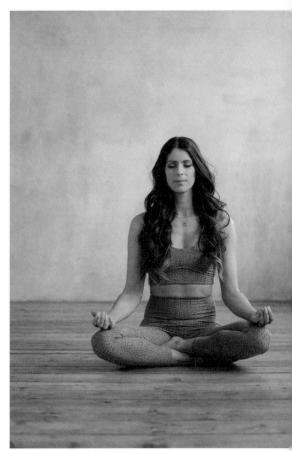

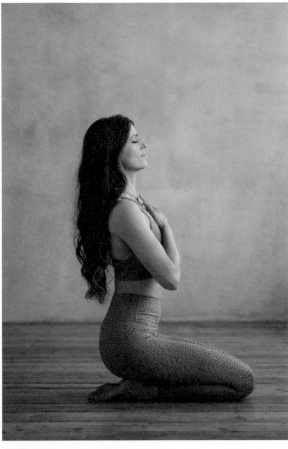

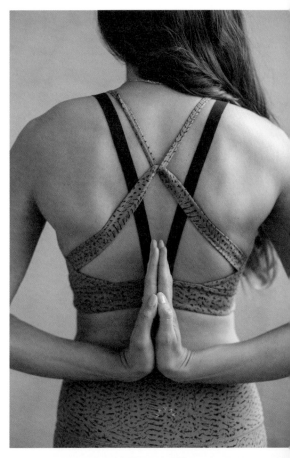

FIND SILENCE

'THE QUIETER YOU BECOME,
THE MORE YOU CAN HEAR.'

RAM DASS

I used to think that meditation was just for hippies. I had a job in finance working all hours and was so busy I thought, 'I don't have time for that!' It seemed counterintuitive to prioritise a time to be still when there were so many things to do. However, once I actually tried it and then introduced a daily meditation practice, I began to notice that taking 10 minutes or so to sit and be still had a positive impact on my whole day. I was *more* productive, *more* connected and *more* creative. Not only that but I was calmer and less reactive to situations.

This doesn't mean I found it easy; quite the opposite. When I began to sit quietly, the internal chatter often became unbearable. But over time calm came and with this, the chance to notice the subtle and generally to see things more clearly. Meditation is not simply sitting down and doing nothing; it's training the mind to increase awareness.

I urge you to read this chapter with curiosity, particularly if meditation and finding silence feels really foreign or something you 'don't have time for'. Thinking back to my old job as an actuary, with hindsight and my yoga training I *know* the huge benefit I would have seen from prioritising the time for meditation. When we get 'too busy' sometimes we *need* to take a step back, have a pause, hit 'reset' and see the bigger picture. We are all 'too busy', but set an intention to give some of the practices at the end of this chapter a try and notice the impact they have on your mind and to your life.

'MEDITATION IS A DANCE
BETWEEN THE THOUGHTS THAT
COME IN AND YOUR ANCHOR
BACK TO THE PRESENT MOMENT.'

MAHATMA GANDHI

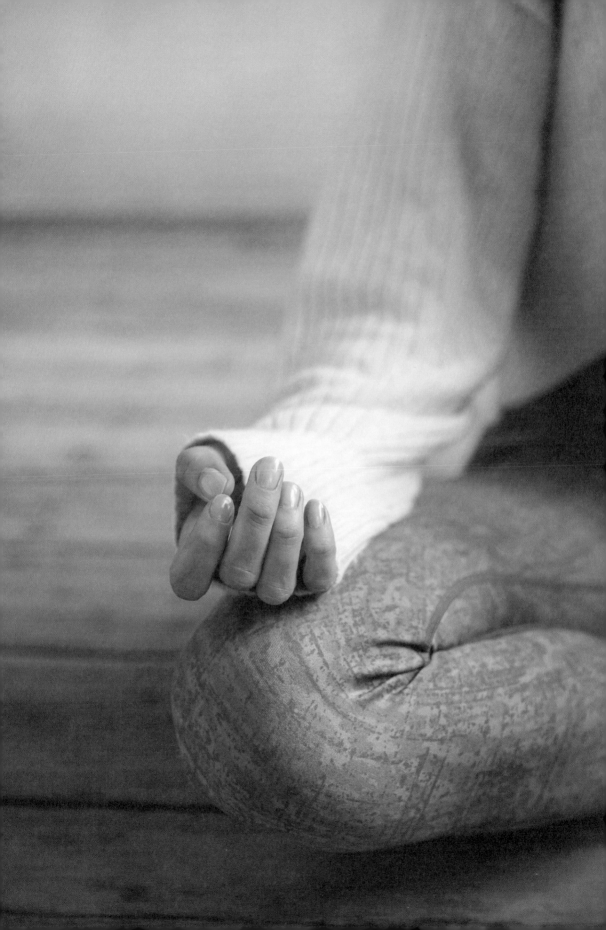

QUIETEN THE NOISE

In our increasingly complex, messy world, meditation is needed more than ever to help us tune out all the noise even for just a moment, and the simple reason is stress. Whether it's anxiety, depression, eating disorders, insomnia, digestive issues, chronic fatigue or just feeling like the world is out of control with so much negative news, many people feel overwhelmed and overloaded. Technology has become intertwined with all aspects of our lives and we are being constantly stimulated in some way throughout all hours of the day.

During the coronavirus pandemic of 2020 I caught Covid-19 and it knocked me for six. It took me a month to recover and during this time my anxiety levels were at an all-time high. I was terrified that people I loved would get ill too and worried what would happen if they did. Social media and the news became something that filled me with dread.

The tools from my yoga practice saved me, and meditation played a huge part in reining in the anxiety. It was at this point that I upped my meditation practice to 40 minutes a day and it wasn't easy. At first the quiet felt like a breeding ground for intrusive thoughts and anxieties.

Over time however it gave me so much insight into my thoughts and I began not only to look forward to the moments of silence but the impact they had on my anxiety, clarity and happiness during the day.

Being busy all the time can hinder productivity and leaves no room for reflection – there's a reason why some of the world's most successful people swear by meditation. If you find yourself constantly doing, and never take time to stop and be, meditation could be a valuable tool in your life.

Many of us fear sitting still and being in the moment, but if we are constantly on the go we risk never taking a moment to appreciate and look at how far we've come or the beauty in what is surrounding us in the moment, right here and now.

In our noisy world, it's important we remember how to turn down the volume both in and outside our heads. It is simply one of our best defences to keep ourselves strong.

'MEDITATION PRACTICE ISN'T ABOUT TRYING TO THROW OURSELVES AWAY AND BECOME SOMETHING BETTER. IT'S ABOUT BEFRIENDING WHO WE ALREADY ARE.'

PEMA CHÖDRÖN

THE BENEFITS OF MEDITATION

Do you find yourself having a short fuse, losing your temper often and then regretting it afterwards? Or perhaps you suffer from insomnia or other sleeping issues – struggling to get to sleep, stay asleep and/or get a quality night's rest? Maybe for you, anxiety is the issue. In 2018 a UK Mental Health Foundation study found that 74 per cent of people have become so stressed they have felt overwhelmed or unable to cope.

Research has shown a multitude of benefits of meditation including that it may improve immunity, help control pain, improve sleep quality, enhance self-awareness and self-esteem and, of course, reduce stress and anxiety.

Whatever it is that you're struggling with or that you may want a stronger handle on, I'd suggest you give meditation a try. It's an ancient practice that has worked for millions of people and in modern life is needed more than ever.

It is worth noting, however, that while meditation brings numerous positive benefits for many, it may not work for all. For people who have experienced trauma or a painful life event, sitting quietly can be difficult and even painful. If you find that meditation brings up more than you feel you can deal with, please speak to a trusted health professional.

THE REWARDS OF A REGULAR MEDITATION PRACTICE

▶ Reduced stress and anxiety

▶ Enhanced self-awareness

▶ Improved sleep quality

▶ Encourages a healthy lifestyle

▶ May slow ageing (both mind and body)

▶ Improved immunity

▶ Encourages better control of unhelpful habits e.g. stress eating, nail biting (i.e. by employing mindfulness)

▶ Improved self-efficacy (and self-esteem)

▶ Decreased blood pressure

▶ Improved problem-solving abilities

▶ Can help control pain

MINDFULNESS VS MEDITATION; WHAT'S THE DIFFERENCE?

Mindfulness is a practice that can occur in every aspect of our lives and involves cultivating a present moment awareness that has no judgement. Thoughts, sensations and feelings come and go and we can mindfully witness them all without allowing them to cloud and consume our thought processes. When you are practising mindfulness, you are paying attention to the world around you, to your thoughts, your feelings, the way you behave, the way you move and the effect you have on those around you.

The idea of mindfulness often conjures up someone with a lot of time, maybe walking through nature drinking in everything around them with full awareness. But mindfulness can work in every aspect of life. Whatever your job is, practise mindfulness by being fully present with your work. Keep your attention focused but alert so as to take on any situation that should arise. Mindfulness also links in with the breath as the breath is an invaluable tool to anchor you to the present, so when you feel your attention drifting, use your breath as a tool to bring it back.

The person that you are today is shaped by the experiences of your past. These past experiences can have an unconscious influence over your thoughts, behaviour and emotions. Think about how much of your day happens automatically, almost like you're on autopilot. Even conscious choices are shaped by the experiences of our past. By being able to observe ourselves regularly and more closely, with mindfulness we can have greater self-control and self-awareness. This will help us make better choices and take control of reactions and their consequences.

I read a beautiful book on mindfulness by spiritual leader Thích Nhat Hanh called *The Miracle of Mindfulness*. The book talks about practising mindfulness every minute, every hour of every day. In reality, this is difficult, so it then goes on to talk about setting one day per week aside for mindfulness; say that every Sunday you know that this is your mindfulness day and you do every single activity keeping your attention focused, keeping anchored to the present moment.

As you wake you are mindful of your morning routine, you take each part slowly, you pay full attention. Even as you wash your body you are doing so mindfully. I personally think this is a beautiful concept and I'm trying to bring it into my life – and know that over time this mindfulness day will slowly turn into a mindfulness week. Opposite is a list of daily activities – can you bring mindfulness into each them? For example, when you're washing your hair, take time to feel the water on your skin; notice the smell of the shampoo and enjoy the sensation of massaging your scalp.

Harvard University psychologists Matthew A Killingsworth and Daniel T Gilbert undertook a study that found that people spend nearly 47 per cent of their waking hours thinking about something other than what they're doing, and that this typically makes them unhappy. Killingsworth says, 'Mind-wandering is an excellent predictor of people's happiness. In fact, how often our minds leave the present and where they tend to go is a better predictor of our happiness than the activities in which we are engaged.' So start to introduce more mindfulness into your day, whether that is through a full day of mindfulness or just bringing mindfulness into certain tasks, such as the ideas opposite.

While mindfulness and meditation have some connections, they are not the same thing. Meditation is a form of mindfulness, but mindfulness is not necessarily meditation.

Research has shown meditation to be effective in helping people be more mindful in their daily life. There are many types of meditation, and different techniques have different qualities and can bring with it different results. For example, a loving kindness meditation focuses on cultivating love and kindness for ourselves and for others, whereas a three-minute breath focused meditation can create calm for times when you are feeling stressed and anxious.

BRING MORE MINDFULNESS INTO EVERYDAY LIFE

▶ Brushing your teeth

▶ Washing your hair

▶ Eat meals with awareness

▶ Travelling to work

▶ Drinking a cup of tea

▶ Mindful interactions: undivided attention

▶ Gardening

▶ Eating chocolate

▶ Mindful walking

▶ Listening to music

▶ Practise meditation

▶ Flow on your mat

▶ Question your urges (e.g. social media scrolling or food binges)

HOW MINDFULNESS WORKS

I watched an interview recently between meditation and mindfulness expert, Maude Hirst, and neuroscientist Dr Tamara Russell. Tamara was explaining how mindfulness actually works and the neural and cognitive processes that are engaged while we practise it. Whilst this sounds complicated, she explains it in a clear, simple and easy to understand way. I am someone who, particularly at the beginning of my yoga journey, had the most runaway mind during mindfulness and meditation so the way Tamara explains mindfulness below really resonated with me. I subsequently had a call with Tamara and bought her amazing book, *What Is Mindfulness?* and she kindly agreed to let me share some of her research and thoughts.

Tamara teaches mindfulness using the following neurocognitive model which recognises that there are four brain states of mindfulness and helps to explain the mindfulness process:

1. Paying attention to the present moment.

2. Becoming distracted (lost in the future or past).

3. Noticing that your mind has wandered.

4. Refocusing your attention back to the present moment.

Once we recognise that these four stages exist, it helps us to realise that it's unrealistic to assume we can live in a constant state of presence, which is sometimes how mindfulness can be misconstrued. Mind-wandering is in fact part of the process of mindfulness, recognising it and bringing your attention back to step one is the essence of mindfulness.

Tamara goes on to explain that there are two other key concepts that underpin these four stages:

▸ INTENTION Knowing what you are doing and why (for example, you want to become less emotionally reactive or create more focus in your day-to-day life).

▸ SELF-COMPASSION Knowing that your mind will wander and that's okay and remembering the intention.

So why does this model work really well? Firstly, it normalises and gives permission for people's minds to wander. This gives immediate relief to those of us with busy minds and let's us know that it's *normal* to have a wandering mind. It also allows people to know that mindfulness is a circular process. People can think, 'where am I in the model?' which helps them know what to do next.

Having an underlying intention for your mindfulness practice reinforces what you are trying to do and gives your brain a compass so that you can bring it back to paying attention to the present moment (otherwise you could get stuck in the mind-wandering phase, with nothing to drive you back towards refocusing your attention). The element of self-compassion then comes in reminding us gently why we are doing this, which is really the heart of mindfulness. Our learning and development will be easier if we are kind to ourselves while practising.

Being aware of these four steps and practising them means that you'll become more and more familiar with the process. Over time the loop will get smaller and smaller and you will become less distracted and be able to focus your attention for longer.

THE FOUR-STEP 'MINDFUL MOMENT' CYCLE

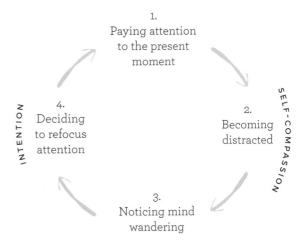

'MINDFULNESS PROVIDES THE TOOLS TO ALLOW YOU TO USE YOUR MIND FLEXIBLY AND TO ITS BEST POTENTIAL, WHETHER YOU'RE MEDITATING, CREATING OR RELATING TO OTHERS. IT IS THE BUILDING BLOCK THAT ALLOWS YOU TO DO ANY OF THESE THINGS, ONLY BETTER.'

DR TAMARA RUSSELL

HOW ARE MEDITATION AND YOGA LINKED?

Have you ever noticed that if you focus your attention fully on only one thing, everything else around you seems to fade? *Pratyahara* is the fifth limb of yoga and is the act of withdrawing the mind from the senses towards the core of your being. Once your awareness turns inwards, your attention is focused and external distractions evaporate.

Dharana and *dhyana* are the sixth and seventh limbs of yoga and they work to discipline the mind on our journey towards freedom. *Dharana* is often referred to as meditation but it is in fact concentration – the observation of a single object, spot, place within or outside the body – in the mind. You can think of it as training the mind; setting it up for meditation. During *asana* we may often use the breath as this object of concentration focusing on its sound, rhythm, depth and quality. Other objects used are a flame, a person or a mantra but what you choose to focus on can be anything.

When we practise concentration, we do it without judgement. The aim is to avoid comparing or measuring the object of our concentration against anything else. Although this isn't a typical practice of *dharana*, I like to do this with my children, say when I am watching them in the garden playing together. Can I be fully present, taking in every moment, avoiding all the things trying to catch my attention and distract me?

Dhyana translates as meditation and continuous focus. There are so many different interpretations of what meditation is and what it should be. Some

people believe that as concentration on an object develops it becomes steadier and unwavering, which means we have entered into the state of meditation. Others believe that meditation doesn't require an object. They believe the object is gone and unwavering focus remains; a sense of being, no judgement, comparison or measurement.

On pages 94–97 I share a number of my favourite meditation techniques for you to try. I recommend trying each of them and seeing which style resonates with you the most – this may depend on your mood or what you need that day.

Over time, focus will become unwavering and *dharana* will become *dhyana*. You'll sit down to meditate for 20 minutes and the timer will go off after what seems like 20 seconds. You may also see visions, hear sounds or be overcome by a particular emotion. It brings us one step closer to *samadhi*, the eighth limb of yoga – complete attention and being in oneness with the universe.

Through the practice of yoga and the different techniques it teaches, we gain awareness and connection. If you can't take the awareness yoga instills in you off the mat and into your daily life, you aren't going to fully reap the benefits. (This isn't just achieved through the physical practice; one must accept every part of yoga – meditation, breath work and the *yamas* and *niyamas* as well). Sometimes we can forget that things like breath work and meditation take time and practice just like *asana* does. You would never expect to walk up to a yoga mat for the first time, place your hands down and float up into a handstand.

Equally, you are never going to sit for the first time and experience a magical stilling of your mind. In some ways, meditation can be harder than practising *asana* as we are so used to always being on the go. It can work wonders but you have to give it time. Meditation is hard and the vast majority of people who try to meditate will give up and move on. Be consistent in a daily practice and you'll start to notice how it has a positive impact on your whole life.

YOGA NIDRA

Yoga *nidra*, also known as 'yogic sleep', is a form of guided meditation which you practise lying down in *savasana* (see page 169). The practice draws our focus inwards towards a natural state of equilibrium and promotes deep rest and relaxation on a physical, mental and emotional level.

In terms of Patañjali's *Yoga Sūtras*, yoga *nidra* would be the limbs *pratyahara* (sense withdrawal), *dharana* (concentration) and *dhyana* (meditation). A yoga *nidra* guided meditation is designed to take you into the state of conscious deep sleep with the mind still awake. You could think of this as the state between being awake and being asleep. When I have had issues with insomnia in the past, yoga *nidra* has been such a saviour.

WHAT ACTUALLY HAPPENS WHEN WE MEDITATE?

When we are stressed our sympathetic nervous system (our 'fight or flight' system) is activated, setting off many reactions in the body including the release of stress chemicals such as cortisol and adrenaline, a spike in our immune system, rise in heart rate and blood pressure, increased perspiration, narrowed focus of attention and shutdown of our digestive system. Back in prehistoric times when we were being chased by a sabre tooth tiger, this response was really useful. By increasing the heart rate and redirecting blood flow and energy from the digestive system and immune function to our limbs, we could battle the sabre tooth tiger or run away.

The problem is the world has evolved so much since prehistoric times but our stress response has not. We are hit by stress from all angles daily – whether through overwork, pressure at home or the negative stories surrounding us on the news and social media. The stresses in our modern lives have increased enormously and look *very* different to what they would have looked like in ancient times, but our body still responds in the same way. We can't just turn this reflex off and our stress response isn't helpful to modern day pressures.

Meditation helps to activate that all-important parasympathetic nervous system – our 'rest-and-digest' system. It helps to turn off our stress response and bring us back into balance. It slows down the heart rate, breathing rate and blood pressure, and soothes the other sympathetic nervous system fight or flight responses.

A number of scientific research studies have shown that meditation can change the structure and function of critical areas of the brain, help relieve anxieties, and boost focus and compassion. A study by Luders, Charbuin and Kurth found that long-term meditators had more grey matter volume in their brain than non-meditators. Grey matter includes regions of the brain involved in moving muscles, hearing, speech and decision-making. It decreases with age.

When we are overwhelmed by thoughts and emotions, it's important to remember that these feelings don't last 100 per cent of the time; we are ever changing. I used to suffer badly from lack of self-belief, never thinking I was good enough and always finding my flaws. That negative thought process was essentially a bad habit.

Think about when you learn a new yoga posture; we train our brain to move in a certain way, forming neural pathways that over time make the movements easier. The same is true for the mind. Meditation can help form new neural pathways, ridding us of those old habits that don't serve our happiness.

Meditation helped me step back and recognise that I am not my thoughts and the impact they were having on me. In turn this helped rid me of my lack of self-belief.

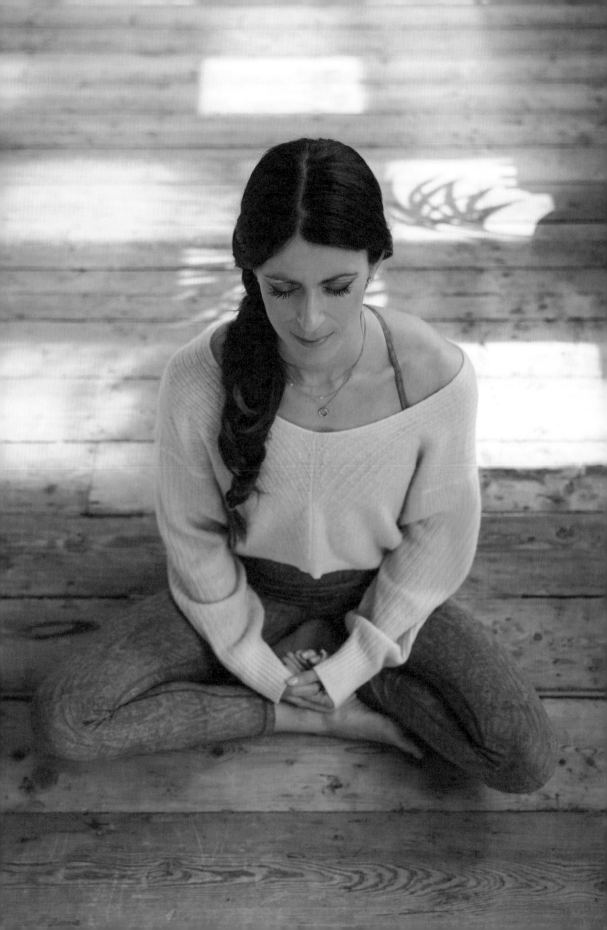

HOW TO MAKE MEDITATION A HABIT

▶ **FIND A MOTIVE**
Before you start on this journey of bringing meditation into your life, take a moment to jot down *why* you want to do it. Whether it's to achieve enlightenment or just to have some added mental focus, *what* the final aim is doesn't matter – have no judgement for it – but the motivation to get there does. A clear sense of purpose will help to keep you motivated and on track to stick with this new habit.

▶ **TRY MEDITATING FIRST THING**
When you rise, find some time to be still and tune in. It can be helpful to practise before your morning coffee or tea as caffeine can be stimulating and make meditation harder. This was a game changer for me as I now simply set my alarm a little earlier and by the time my children are awake, I feel like I have found some nourishment to put me in a positive mindset to start the day.

▶ **SWITCH IT UP**
Changing location is really helpful to avoid getting too used to meditating in a quiet room. Try meditating on your morning commute or in the park before eating your lunch.

▶ **TRY NEW THINGS**
Meditation can come in many forms and it may be that one isn't right for you at that moment in time. Try different techniques, for example if sitting with the eyes closed isn't right for you, try a walking meditation in nature instead.

▶ **YOUR MIND *WILL* WANDER**
Lots of people try meditation and conclude very quickly it isn't for them as their minds are 'too busy' and forever wandering. However, if you notice that your mind is wandering during your meditation, this kind of means you're doing it right! You've *noticed* that your mind is wandering and therefore can gently bring it back. The more we practise, the easier it becomes, but know that you will still have days where your mind wanders 10, 20, 100 times, and that's okay, you're not doing anything wrong.

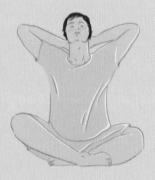
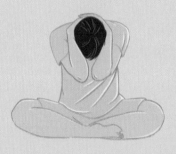
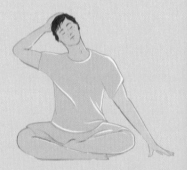

▶ QUICK MEDITATION BREAK

If you don't have a lot of time, a five-minute meditation break to hit pause and get a little mental recharge can be so valuable.

▶ GET COMFORTABLE!

For most of us, sitting on a hard floor in lotus pose isn't going to be comfortable and will make meditation harder. Instead, find a comfortable seat; this can be a sofa or a chair with an upright back. Before you begin, make sure you are comfortable and supported, with the head, neck and back aligned, and shoulders relaxed.

▶ BREATHE NATURALLY

Although meditation is often focused on the breath to help anchor you to the now, don't try and change it in any way. Simply be its witness, noticing all sensations and its rhythm.

▶ KNOW THERE WILL BE DISCOMFORT

Uncomfortable feelings like frustration and anxiety can frequently appear during meditation. When we tune in and pay attention, truths can be uncovered that were previously buried. Sit with these feelings and sensations, don't try and brush them aside. Simply breathe into them and give them awareness without judgement, allowing them to come and go. Know that you always have the choice to stop if it becomes too uncomfortable.

▶ CHECK IN

After each meditation jot down how you felt before and afterwards. Avoid labels such as 'good' or 'bad' and instead note how you are feeling physically, emotionally and mentally.

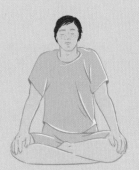
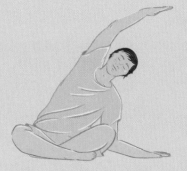
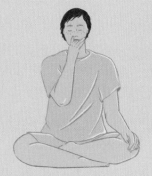

MEDITATION TECHNIQUES

In a study published in the *European Journal of Social Psychology* in 2009, health psychology researcher Phillippa Lally states that it takes 66 days to develop a habit. So, I challenge you for the next 66 days to bring meditation into your life, even if that is five minutes every morning.

Try a couple of the techniques that follow to see what works for you. Know there will be days where it feels almost impossible (that's okay, it happens to me a lot!) but other days where it will feel amazing. It's an up and down journey. But what you will develop is a lifelong tool to help you weather the storm we call life.

The four different meditation techniques can be used daily. They are my favourite types of meditation and I think that they complement each other well. I find myself using them all depending on how I am feeling or what I need. I would recommend trying one technique each day for 10 minutes or more, but remember, if you are struggling for time then five minutes is better than nothing.

WALKING MEDITATION

A moving meditation connects body and breath by bringing awareness to all sensations using simple movements to anchor you in the present. I am sharing a simple walking meditation here but in essence it can be any movement you like. Be mindful of all sensations, the feeling of your breath, any tension or discomfort, the effect of the movements on your mind and body; be open to them all.

We can so often walk (like we breathe) on autopilot. In a walking meditation you focus the attention fully on the sensations in the soles of your feet or the sensations in the muscles and joints of the legs. The best location to practise is outdoors; a back garden or park, or even a quiet pavement. Choose a place where you won't be interrupted and where you don't need to make decisions as to where you walk.

Start with a 15-minute practice and gradually build up to 30 minutes to an hour.

Directions:
▶ As you walk, bring your full focus into the present moment. Walk at a regular pace observing the change in sensations in the feet as you walk.

▶ Feel free to intentionally move your attention to any sounds, objects and smells, but the key is intention. Intentionally allow the mind to explore and observe them.

SEATED MEDITATIONS

For the following meditations, come into a comfortable seated position with a straight back. You may like to sit on the floor or on a chair with an upright back, whichever is most comfortable for you. Push down into the chair/floor and find length in the spine.

Gently close your eyes, keeping your gaze lowered to keep your forehead soft. If you don't like to close your eyes, you can have the eyes slightly open with the gaze lowered to the floor in front of you.

Close your lips and let your breath come in and out through the nose in its natural rhythm.

Before each meditation begins, it can be nice to feel your sitting bones on the chair and your feet on the floor. Imagine roots winding down from these areas, helping you feel secure and grounded.

After each meditation session take a moment to reflect and jot down how it made you feel and anything of note that came up (if the answer is nothing then that's okay too!).

BREATHING MEDITATION

Our breath keeps us here in the present moment. By using the breath as the main focus of this meditation, it acts as an anchor to the now by bringing your awareness to all sensations of the breath, allowing the mind to settle.

Directions:

▶ Come into a comfortable seated position, somewhere where you can be free of distractions.

▶ Set a timer for 5–20 minutes.

▶ Take a few deep breaths in through the nose and out through the mouth. Feel the earth beneath your sitting bones and under your feet and notice how this provides a sense of feeling grounded and settled.

▶ Release control of the breath and simply start to watch it. Notice how each breath looks different, how various parts of your body move as you breathe. Notice the slight pause between each inhale and exhale, exhale and inhale. Notice any sounds the breath makes, notice *every* sensation that each breath brings.

▶ Each time your mind starts to wander, gently bring your awareness back to your breath and the present moment.

▶ When the timer finishes, take a moment with the eyes still closed to sit and notice how you feel and any thoughts or feelings that arose.

MANTRA MEDITATION

A mantra is a phrase you repeat to yourself, typically composed of only a few words or syllables. The meaning of mantra is 'that which keeps the mind steady and produces the proper effect'. I have offered three different mantras that you can use for this meditation below but feel free to use your own if you prefer.

Possible mantras:

▶ 'Aum' or 'Om' – a sacred sound known as the sound of the universe. Om is meant to activate the third eye and crown *chakras* (see page 41), allowing us connect to our true selves.

▶ 'So Hum' – in Sanskrit this translates to mean 'I am'. This mantra is good at balancing the root *chakra* (see page 40) and will help you to connect within and find self-love.

▶ 'In me, I trust' – a mantra that I love because it's a gentle reminder to go within and trust that we have the answers and don't need to turn outwards for them.

Directions:

▶ Come into a comfortable seated position, somewhere you can be free of distractions.

▶ Set a timer for 5-20 minutes.

▶ Take a few deep breaths in through the nose and out through the mouth. Feel the earth beneath your sit bones and under your feet and notice how this provides a sense of feeling grounded and settled.

▶ Start to silently repeat your chosen mantra, slowly, softly like you're whispering it within your body.

▶ Each time your mind starts to wander, gently bring your awareness back to your mantra.

▶ When the timer finishes, take a moment with the eyes still closed to sit and notice how you feel and any thoughts or feelings that arose.

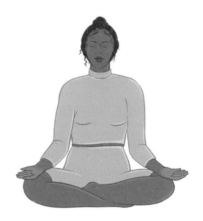

LOVING-KINDNESS MEDITATION

Loving-kindness meditations and compassion meditations are important components of mindfulness. Developing and cultivating our ability to show ourselves and others kindness and compassion can help to improve our own happiness, confidence and mental health. With kindness and compassion, we can respond more positively to unpleasant and negative events and emotions. It also helps us to overcome the illusion of being totally separate from others and we can start to think about the connection between us all.

The meditation is based around the following affirmations/mantras:

▸ May all beings be safe and free from suffering.

▸ May all beings be peaceful.

▸ May all beings be filled with loving-kindness.

▸ May all beings accept themselves just as they are.

Directions:

▸ Come into a comfortable seated position, somewhere where you can be free of distractions.

▸ Set a timer for 10–20 minutes.

▸ Take a few deep breaths in through the nose and out through the mouth. Feel the earth beneath your sitting bones and under your feet and notice how this provides a sense of feeling grounded and settled.

▸ Now start to silently bring yourself feelings of kindness, similar to those you would give to a loved one. We all have the same feelings of inadequacy, we can all make mistakes, we are all human. Start to slowly and silently repeat to yourself two to three times (or more): 'May I be safe and free from suffering, may I be peaceful, may I be filled with loving-kindness, may I accept myself just as I am.'

▸ Now slowly start to bring to mind a loved one. Silently share this kindness and compassion with them two to three times (or more): 'May you be safe and free from suffering, may you be peaceful, may you be filled with loving-kindness, may you accept yourself just as you are.'

▸ Now slowly start to bring to mind someone who you perhaps find a little more difficult, who you don't get on with as well. Silently share this kindness and compassion with them two to three times (or more): 'May you be safe and free from suffering, may you be peaceful, may you be filled with loving-kindness, may you accept yourself just as you are.'

▸ Now bring to mind all beings, everywhere; let's share this loving-kindness with everyone. Silently repeat two to three times (or more): 'May all beings be safe and free from suffering, may all beings be peaceful, may all beings be filled with loving-kindness, may all beings accept themselves just as they are.'

▸ Each time your mind starts to wander, gently bring your awareness back to the present moment.

▸ When the timer finishes, take a moment with the eyes still closed to sit and notice how you feel and any thoughts or feelings that arose.

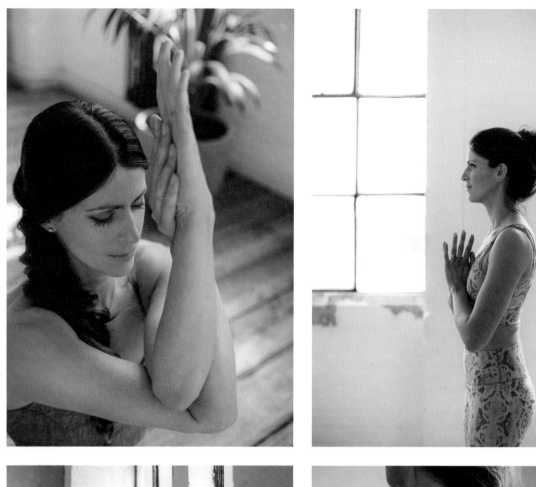
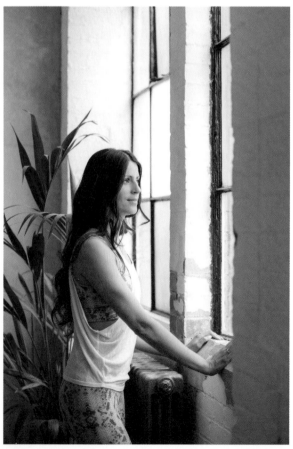
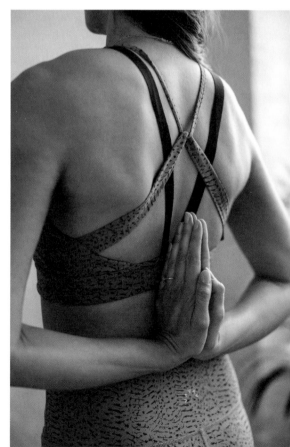

THE POWER OF YOUR WORDS

'KIND WORDS CAN BE SHORT
AND EASY TO SPEAK, BUT THEIR
ECHOES ARE TRULY ENDLESS.'

MOTHER TERESA

How we speak to others and how we speak to ourselves can have immense power. In essence, our thoughts, the words we speak and how we absorb the words of others controls the reality we live in. One of the things I spend a lot of time doing as a teacher is preparing yoga classes with themes that will speak to my students both on and off the mat. I can't tell you how many times I've seen students moved to tears (me included) by the theme and wording interlaced throughout a yoga class. As we have already seen, a yoga class isn't just about linking postures together; it's about finding connection within, learning more about yourself and finding kindness and compassion towards yourself and others – the goal being to help you to lead a calm, happy and more holistic life. The words spoken during a practice both out loud and internally matter.

In this chapter I will help you understand the power in words – not just in the words we say to others, but in our internal dialogue too. I will outline techniques to help you develop more mindfulness around words and I will lead you through the setting of intentions and affirmations so that you can learn how to take charge of your thoughts and change your thinking patterns to help transform your life.

'HAPPINESS IS WHEN WHAT YOU THINK, WHAT YOU SAY, AND WHAT YOU DO ARE IN HARMONY.'

MAHATMA GANDHI

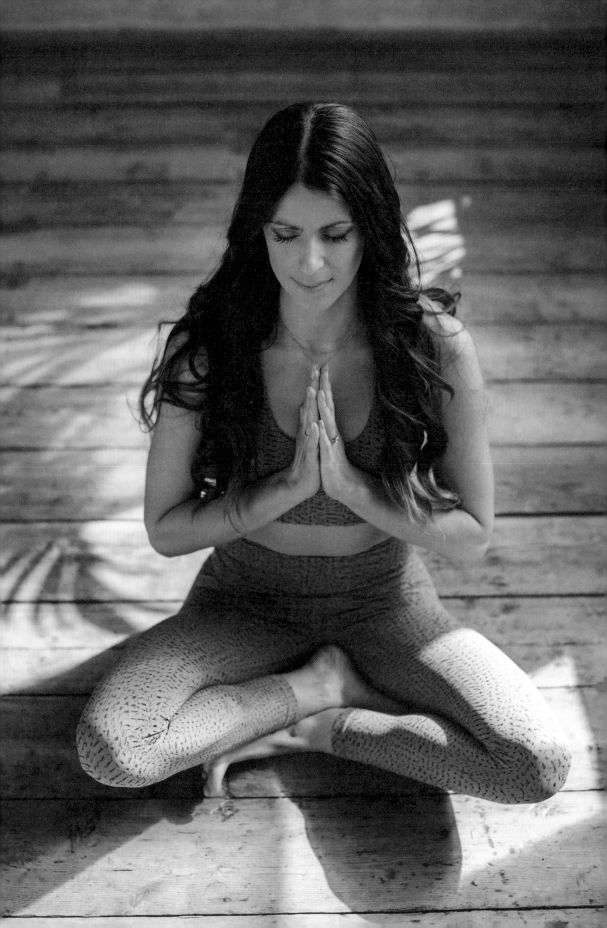

THE POWER OF
OUR INTERNAL DIALOGUE

Your 'inner dialogue' is, simply put, your thoughts. That voice inside that comments on your life, consciously and subconsciously. Yoga helps us recognise our thoughts, find patterns or habits, and study them in order to create freedom from them and thrive in life on all levels.

The fourth *niyama* is *svadhyaya* or 'self-study' (see page 136) and it's about knowing our true identity. In the book *The Yamas and Niyamas* by Deborah Adele, Deborah describes human beings as a diamond ring wrapped in many boxes or layers. These layers are born from our personal experience: our childhood, education, affluence, where we are born and so on, all feed into them. *Svadhyaya* helps us to understand these layers.

Yoga reminds us that we are the core, not these layers, and part of the idea of self-study is to remind us of our true identity. It helps us understand our layers and why they are there. Doing this in turn helps us to understand why we act or react in a certain way. For example, if your childhood lacked compassion and you were punished for every mistake you made, you may still carry around this experience.

When you or others make a mistake your mind immediately thinks punishment whereas we are human, we make mistakes and punishment shouldn't be the immediate nor only reaction. We can treat mistakes with empathy, compassion and understanding. There's a beautiful quote from a poem by thirteenth century Persian poet Rumi that says: 'Raise your words, not voice. It is rain that grows flowers, not thunder.'

We dive more into this in on pages 114–121 but self-study is a useful concept to keep in mind when we consider the words we think and speak and why certain habits or thought patterns may occur.

In establishing your yoga practice, both on and off the mat, you need to support yourself through positive self-talk, compassion and understanding. This will make it easier to sustain a yoga habit.

If we think of some of the *yamas* we have talked about already (see page 126), they remind us of this. For example, *ahimsa* (or non-violence) and finding kindness towards yourself; knowing that maintaining a yoga habit in this modern world is difficult and having empathy for yourself if you're finding the physical practice challenging, or if you only have three minutes today to stop and breathe.

Satya is truthfulness and can be reflected in a yoga plan that is realistic. How many times have you intended to squeeze everything into your day, allowing no time for breaks or things to come in that weren't expected? This can result in a sense of failure if we don't get everything done that we have intended to. In reality, if we had just been truthful and realistic with ourselves at the start of the day, we could have felt the opposite way. So, when you are thinking of a yoga plan, find truth and realistic expectations.

When your inner dialogue is filled with negativity and you continually beat yourself up for even the smallest of infractions, it creates unrest inside you. When I learned how to flip my perspective and change the way I spoke to myself, challenging those negative thoughts and replacing them with kindness, it changed me as a person.

This isn't just a 'fake it 'til you make it' mentality. It's not about pretending everything is absolutely amazing (this, too, can result in inner turmoil). It's more about recognising negative thoughts and feelings and reminding yourself that you have the power to rewrite the narrative and reframe your thoughts. We need to be reminded of what is positive, not just within ourselves, but all around us so that we have the tools to cope when things aren't so easy.

One thing that has been transformational for me over the past few years is giving myself the love, respect and compassion I would give to a friend (again relating back to *ahimsa* and non-violence). Think back to a time when something bad happened – big or small – for which you gave yourself a hard time; perhaps it was forgetting to pick something up, breaking something of value or forgetting a deadline. Think of the way you spoke to yourself, the harsh words you used.

Now think of someone close to you that you love – a partner, a friend, a family member. If they had done the same thing, what would you have said? The answer is probably that you would have had empathy and reminded them that we aren't robots but in fact humans in a deeply chaotic world. Things go wrong, we forget things, we screw up. But if you are constantly putting yourself down for these things, you can't grow. What will help you grow is turning that inner voice around and having some understanding about why it happened, and thinking about how you can stop it happening again.

'I HAVE MET MYSELF AND
I AM GOING TO CARE
FOR HER FIERCELY.'

GLENNON DOYLE

SETTING INTENTIONS

Have you ever been to a yoga class where at the start the teacher tells you to 'set an intention for your practice'? I remember for the first few years of hearing this it actually caused me a little anxiety. I didn't really know what they were asking me to do and there was never any guidance on how to do it.

When I started teaching and delving more into the depths of yoga I realised that in fact it can be very simple. Setting an intention for your practice is bringing your attention to a quality that you would like to achieve both on your yoga mat and in your life.

For example, maybe you are looking for more mindfulness – on the mat you focus on using your breath and body as an anchor to keep you present. You then take this intention off the mat, noticing when your mind wanders and you start running on autopilot, and gently bringing yourself back and finding connection.

Intentions are a powerful tool to help guide a practice and keep your awareness in the now. Your intention can be anything that you want to cultivate: strength, presence, gratitude, awareness of breath – whatever it is you need.

By setting intentions we can actively empower ourselves to make the changes to live the life we desire, and as I mentioned above, intentions in our physical practice are a way of carrying our practice into everyday life. It may be that you decide to wake up each morning and set an intention that you can carry throughout your day. Or instead, maybe you take the theme of the yoga class and make this into an intention – for example a class with a theme of heart opening could carry with it an intention of forgiveness or honesty.

On the opposite page I have set out some of my favourite intentions, which you could use in your own practice. Equally, you should feel free to use an intention that resonates with you and what you're working on. The intention you choose doesn't need to change daily, it could even stick with you over the month or a few months. Don't rush in choosing it – take time to breathe, listen within and bring awareness to a quality that you want to cultivate more of in your life.

If you are asked to set an intention at the start of a yoga class and feel you don't have time to properly think it through, try and come up with something that you can use as a quick fill-in (for me I always come back to an intention of connection). Alternatively, you could choose to dedicate your practice to someone you love, someone who makes you stronger.

An intention should be something that is:

- ▶ Realistic and attainable
- ▶ Short and simple
- ▶ Something you want to cultivate (i.e. rather than 'I don't want to feel like this anymore', it would be 'I have the ability to find strength and ease')

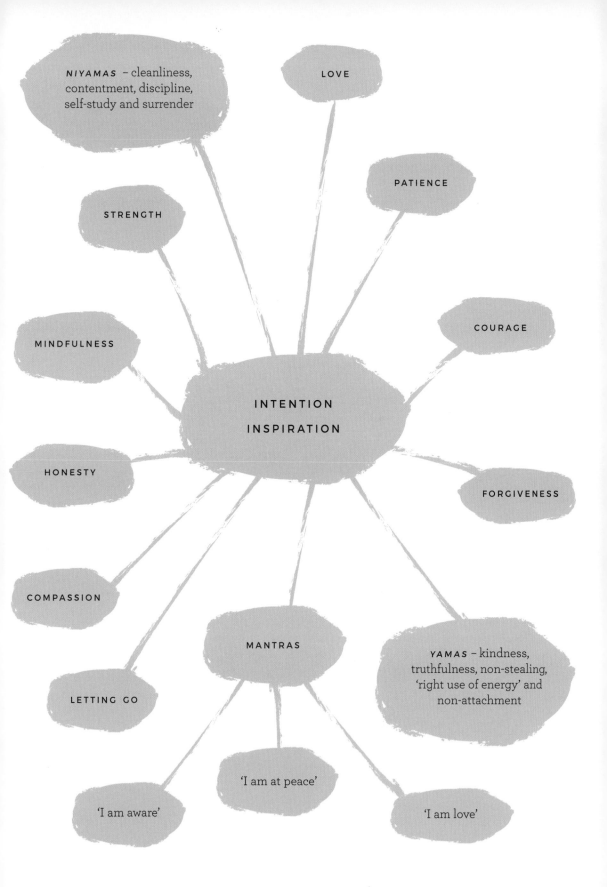

NIYAMAS – cleanliness, contentment, discipline, self-study and surrender

LOVE

PATIENCE

STRENGTH

COURAGE

MINDFULNESS

INTENTION

INSPIRATION

HONESTY

FORGIVENESS

COMPASSION

MANTRAS

YAMAS – kindness, truthfulness, non-stealing, 'right use of energy' and non-attachment

LETTING GO

'I am aware'

'I am at peace'

'I am love'

AFFIRMATIONS

Affirmations are declarations that can help you strengthen the connection between your unconscious and your conscious mind. Affirmations invoke power to create the life you want to live. A famous quote by Buddha says it well: 'You become what you believe.'

Affirmations will influence the way you see yourself and how others see you. Thinking or writing down affirmations allows your brain to focus on the positive, helping you form a positive feeling or emotion. They help you challenge negative thoughts, fears and anxieties and help you realise your full potential. They remind you what you can do and what you can take charge of, rather than leaving you feeling like life is dictating to you.

Some extremely successful people have shouted loudly about the power of affirmations. 'Am I good enough? Yes I am,' wrote former first lady Michelle Obama in her *New York Times* bestselling memoir *Becoming*. American boxing champion Muhammad Ali famously said, 'I am the greatest. I said that even before I knew I was.'

There are two different approaches to introducing affirmations; choose the method you feel would best suit you.

CONSISTENCY Choose one affirmation that really resonates with you and that you want to be a part of your life and write that down every single day or say it silently in your head. This can literally be anything from 'I am strong, I am brave, I am resilient', to 'I am going to make £3,000 a month'. Consistency is my approach, and 98 per cent of the time my affirmation is 'don't sweat the small stuff'. I used to suffer greatly with stress and focusing too much on the 'small stuff', not allowing myself to see the big picture. This affirmation is a constant reminder to me that there are always going to be bumps in the road and I can either let these continually trip me up or remember that life is more than these bumps and I have the power to create my own happiness.

GO WITH THE FLOW Choose an affirmation depending on your current mood, want or plans. Each day it can be something different depending on what you're feeling or working on. For example, if you are working towards a promotion at work it might be 'I am the best person for this role. I am hard-working, committed and fully capable of doing this job.'

When choosing your daily affirmation, here are some top tips:

▸ Start each day by writing it down or saying it out loud. Make it real!

▸ Make it positive.

▸ Think about going to the edge of your comfort zone. If you go too far your affirmation may be something more than you can realistically achieve, and the converse is true; if you chose something that you do already it will be fairly neutral and have minimum impact.

Here are some affirmations I personally love that might resonate with you:

▸ I believe in myself. I believe I can succeed

▸ I choose happiness

▸ I have what it takes to reach my goals

▸ I acknowledge my own self-worth

▸ I face everything with courage

▸ I am dedicated to live in alignment with my purpose

▸ I have strength within me at all times

▸ Don't sweat the small stuff

▸ I will not compare myself to a stranger on the internet

▸ I am enough

▸ I have the power to create change

▸ I can do difficult things

▸ I am living with abundance

▸ I have made mistakes but I will not let them define me

▸ My life has meaning

THE WORDS WE SPEAK

The words we speak out loud define us as individuals and create the reality we live in, whether positive or negative. Words are one of our most powerful tools, therefore let us pick the best words to say, and to hear, in order to create our best reality.

Spend a day watching yourself – imagine it as being a bit like a reality TV show of your life. Be conscious of the words you speak and the tone you use. How do certain things you say make you feel? How do other people react to your words? Can you understand why you say certain things? Do you speak too much?

Recently, my parents' dog Millie died. I was very close to her and my five-year-old son was with me when I found out. It was a really sad but beautiful moment as he just looked at me and could tell I was very upset. He asked what had happened and when I told him, he came over and sat on my lap putting his arms around me. He looked at me and asked why it had happened. I explained she had died simply of old age but then proceeded to tell him story after story of the role Millie had played in my life. He just sat there and listened, without interrupting, giving me the occasional infectious laugh he has.

The reason why it was so beautiful is that often when something sad happens to someone we feel the need to talk, to give advice, to fill the silence. But what yoga teaches us is *asteya* (non-stealing), not stealing the opportunity for someone to talk. To listen – to truly listen – without interruption; without thinking about what we can say to make that person feel better or to share a similar story.

To give that person the opportunity to share and unload.

This leads on to being mindful of your reactions, particularly if someone is showing vulnerability by sharing something hard for them. How you *react* has such power. If you laugh in their face or brush it off as nothing, imagine the impact this has on them. Show others kindness and respect and don't steal their chance to share. This doesn't mean you need to agree with everything others say, but it means that the response you give should be mindful and one that includes compassion and empathy.

One of my wonderful yoga teachers, Lara Heimann, once shared with me this simple reminder based on an ancient philosophy. It links two yogic concepts, *ahimsa* (non-violence) and *satya* (truthfulness), both of which I discuss further on page 28:

Every time you speak ask yourself these three things:

1 IS IT TRUE?
2 IS IT KIND?
3 IS IT NECESSARY?

Speaking the truth sounds easy but what about those slight exaggerations, or when you shape a story to fit a narrative, maybe missing out a part on purpose? Does that still make it true?

The second question is about kindness which can be at odds with the truth. Do you speak words that will cause pain but are true?

The last question can help you decide whether or not to say something/whether or not your words are helpful. We all sometimes avoid saying something that's uncomfortable, but sometimes it is necessary that things are said or, equally, left unsaid.

It is up to you to decide whether your words are going to do good or harm. We are generally aware when we mean to cause harm with our words, but sometimes we say things without first considering the impact they may cause. It's important to become aware of how we speak to one another – particularly given how easy it is with social media to post a hasty comment, or fire off an immediate email response. Come back to the concept of compassion and understanding, even more so if you're upset or angry. Pause to take a deep breath and think about how you're going to respond, whether it's justified and what the other person may be going through. We also need to remember that not all people hear things we say in the same way.

As a child I was often told to 'stop being so sensitive'. This stuck with me for a long time. I tried very hard to bury my emotions in the hope of becoming less sensitive but in reality that made it even worse. Over time I realised that being 'too sensitive' was not a truth I needed in my life. I learnt that feeling isn't a bad a thing; it is, in fact, a form of connection and a form of awareness.

Now instead of feeling bad about being sensitive, I think of it as a quality to be proud of. The point of sharing this story is to show that words can stick with you for years and years. Without the practice of self-study I might not have shaken off this 'belief'. We need to be mindful of the words we speak to others, including our children, because they can have a lasting impact.

The last point I want to make on the power of words is about gossip. We grow up surrounded by it – learnt from friends, parents, magazines, television and social media – and we can grow up thinking it's normal as 'everyone is doing it'.

In his book *The Four Agreements* spiritual teacher Don Miguel Ruiz speaks about gossip being like poison – a way to connect with one another and feel better about ourselves. And if you're truly honest with yourself, think about the last time you gossiped about someone else and how it made you feel. I bet it felt good at first but then afterwards you felt a little muddy, a bit ill at ease.

Use your words only for truth and love and think about the impact they will have on another human being.

ABSORBING THE WORDS OF OTHERS

Mindfulness around words also applies to how we absorb the words of others. One of the very visible and instant sources of judgement and verbal negativity we face today comes from social media. This has started to become a big problem for those who absorb its words viscerally. Even if we are not ourselves the recipients of such negative words, we are witness to them being used towards others. Writing unkind words behind a screen removes an element of accountability and is a lot easier than saying them out loud to someone's face.

In most cases, unkind words are a reflection on the person saying them (and we must reflect on ourselves when we find ourselves rushing to judgement, too). It is important to remember we only know a fraction of what is going on in other people's lives. Also, as much as we may like to think we can influence what other people say, the only thing we can control is how we process their words, any assumptions we try to make and whether we take these words to heart. Learning how to let go of other people's negative words is incredibly freeing. We have choices, including how we react to other people. When someone speaks to us negatively, we can listen, take notice, show compassion and practise empathy – even if we disagree. We can even make the choice to walk away.

Going back to the concept from the start of this chapter about the build-up of layers formed throughout our lives, which shape our reality and experience. Every single one of us has these layers and we don't know what hardships others have suffered. But if someone is holding on to emotional trauma or past abuse, say, or even if they have just had an extremely difficult few weeks or months, this is going to shape their layers. If this person then projects this onto you with their words, it's actually nothing about you. Although their words can be extremely painful, remembering this fact can make it much easier to deal with.

Conversely, most of the things that bother us are indeed a reflection of us, and this, of course, is true for everyone else. So when someone says something that stings, it's a great opportunity for reflection and self-study. Ask yourself, why does this bother me? Where is this stemming from?

THE POWER OF WORDS – TAKEAWAYS

Words impact everything we do and all our interactions. Our days are filled with the words we speak aloud and the thoughts, both conscious and unconscious, that rush around our head.

In many respects that makes this the most important chapter in the book. I therefore thought it would be useful to pull out and remind you of some of the key concepts to help inspire you to change any unwanted habits and transform the ways you think and use your words to interact.

- All words have power whether spoken out loud or internally.

- We are all wrapped in layers born from our personal experiences.

- *Svadhyaya* or 'self-study' helps us to understand these layers and why we react in certain ways.

- Your internal dialogue matters – can you show yourself the kindness and compassion you show others?

- Use intentions to actively empower yourself to make the change you desire.

- Use affirmations to create the life you want to live.

- Be conscious of the words you speak – how do people react to them, how do they make you feel, do you speak too much or too little?

- Ask yourself, 'are these words kind, true and necessary?'

- Give others the opportunity to speak, and be mindful of how you react.

- Beware of gossip; distance yourself from it.

- Others' unkind words are in most cases a reflection on the person saying them and what they are going through.

- When the words of others bother you ask yourself why.

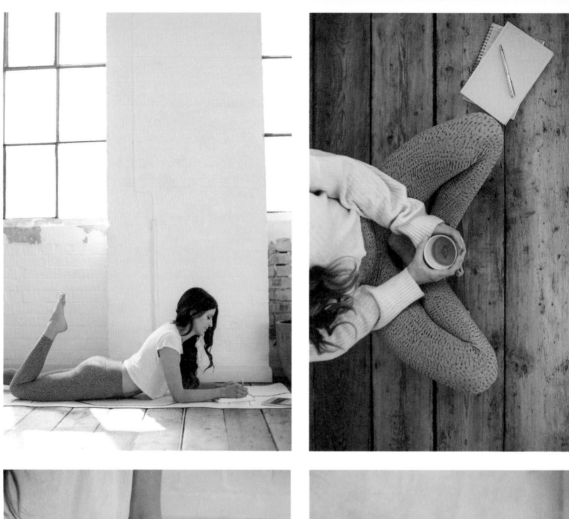

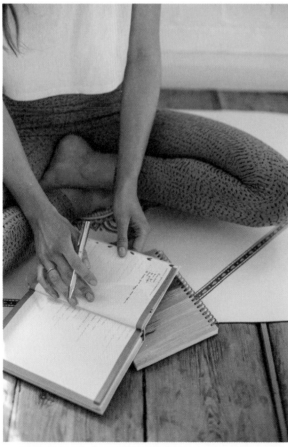

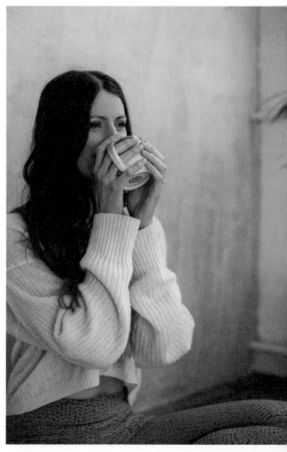

SELF-STUDY

'FILL YOUR PAPER WITH THE
BREATHINGS OF YOUR HEART.'

WILLIAM WORDSWORTH

I didn't keep a journal or diary as a girl, so when I was asked to journal daily as part of my yoga teacher training, it felt uncomfortable, childish and foreign. My tendency towards perfectionism made journaling an initial struggle; I was afraid that I wasn't doing it 'right' and that what I was writing wasn't useful or insightful enough. A part of me also worried that I was going to uncover something from deep inside me that I wouldn't like.

The reality is that there's no right or wrong way to journal and no one is going to judge the way you do it. Ultimately it felt good to unearth the things I uncovered (although sometimes unpleasant), and start the healing process. I can now firmly say that journaling is something I look forward to and I know that it has a positive impact on my life and how connected I feel to myself.

In the previous chapter – The Power of Your Words – we talked about the fourth *niyama*; *svadhyaya*, or 'self-study'. Self-study can be thought of as tuning inwards and reflecting deeply on your practice, thoughts, beliefs and behaviours (it has other applications that I reflect on in the Find Fulfilment and Growth chapter). A wonderful way to approach self-study in order to understand your actions, impressions and the world around you is through journaling and self-reflection. This will guide you to creatively document your thoughts and feelings to help you get to where you want to be – whether or not you think you're creative.

Journaling invites you to look at yourself in an objective and honest way and can bring awareness of both your strengths and limitations. It only needs a few minutes of your day and it doesn't matter what you write – the process of journaling is what's important.

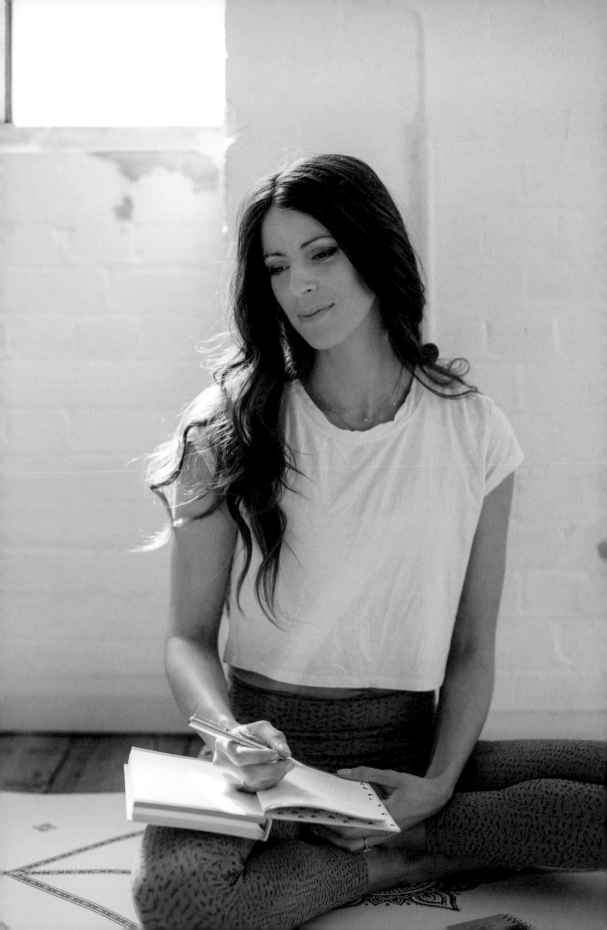

HOW TO JOURNAL

The benefits of journaling and writing down our feelings and worries are well documented but maybe you're thinking where on earth do I start? I like to think about journaling in two stages; stage one is something you write about daily (what are you grateful for, what went well, what you can work on), and stage two is a weekly/bi-weekly self-reflection (digging deeper into habits, behaviours and reactions). I go into these in more detail below.

WHERE TO START

▸ *Short and sweet* – this doesn't need to be something that takes an hour every day. I probably spend a few minutes each morning with my journal and the same before bed. Don't let lack of time hold you back.

▸ *Daily* – be committed to creating a daily journaling habit. Aim to do it at the same time each day and keep your journal in the same place (mine sits on my bedside table). I have found this has the highest success rate for sticking to it and reaping the benefits.

▸ *No fancy journal needed* – although there are some incredible guided journals out there, all you really need is a blank piece of paper, your computer or even an app.

▸ *Plan* – if you know what you are going to write about it can be a lot less daunting than staring at a blank sheet of paper. Guided questions can also help draw out other questions from your mind that you may want to reflect , so on page 119 I have helped you with this.

DAILY PROMPTS

Opposite is a structure that works well for me for the prompts I use in my journal every day. You could spend a couple of minutes each morning and evening on these, or tackle them all at the end of the day or first thing in the morning.

I always refer to this routine as one of my 'happy habits' because they truly do make me happier. Have you ever woken up in the morning to something bad happening – maybe the kids refuse to get dressed or the fridge has broken leaving you with a nightmare you don't have time for? In times like this it is so easy to think 'I'm having an awful day!'. But the only way it's going to be a 'bad day' is if *you* let it. Try and seek out the positives and find gratitude, even if these are smalls things like seeing a friend you love or gratitude for an author of an amazing book you've read. Over time this is going to help you realise that the small things bring so much joy and happiness.

'YOGA IS THE JOURNEY OF THE SELF, THROUGH THE SELF, TO THE SELF.'

THE BHAGAVAD GITA

MORNING PROMPTS:

▶ *Gratitude* – name at least five things you are grateful for, avoiding repetition day to day as much as possible. There are many studies that show the power of gratitude and how it can make you happier, less stressed, improve your physical health and enhance empathy (amongst other things).

▶ *Affirmation* – write an affirmation down daily and use it to help you find power to create the life you want to live (see pages 106–107 for how to set affirmations).

▶ *Two goals* – write down two things you want to achieve in your day. This can, of course, be more but I always have the intention of just getting two things done. It goes back to the principle of *satya* (truthfulness) and having realistic, achievable goals.

EVENING PROMPTS:

▶ *Five positives* – what five positive things happened in your day? If this feels like a struggle or if you've had a really difficult day, keep it simple. For example, include things like 'had a nice meal', 'took a warm shower' or even 'made the bed'.

▶ *What could have gone better?* – here's your chance to reflect on what didn't serve you and what you want to change. Take a moment to reflect on anything that caused you or others some level of anguish, and what you can do tomorrow to help avoid this happening. This isn't an opportunity to beat yourself up or feel like a failure – in fact it's the opposite. Recognising something doesn't serve you but actively setting an intention on how to change this is a step forward, not a step back.

These simple prompts can help you realise that even on the dark days, you have more resilience and solutions than you give yourself credit for. They remind you that you are the author of your story and with this you hold the power of choice. Choose strength, choose seeing the light through the clouds, choose finding happiness.

SELF-REFLECTION

This is the part of journaling that can be more difficult and takes a little more thought and soul searching. I try and sit down for at least 10 minutes a week and work my way through four questions (or more) like the ones I have set out opposite. Alternatively, you could contemplate one of these questions each day.

Find a quiet space where you won't be disturbed and consider making it into a treat, for example, have a mug of your favourite tea and light a scented candle – the more you look forward to journaling, the easier it is to form a habit.

When you go through the questions, try not to overthink; write from the heart and see what you uncover. This exercise of self-reflection is about nourishing the inner voice and questioning it. Why do you react in certain ways or think certain things? What are the things in your life that sustain and drain you? Where do your passions lie and where do you want to succeed in life?

The questions can open doors and help you recognise parts of life where you are spending unnecessary energy, and others where you need to spend more. I have included a number of starter questions opposite; start by picking the questions that resonate immediately.

Over time, when journaling becomes a habit, direct yourself back to the ones you have avoided. Ask yourself why you've avoided them, dive in and go for it.

Another way of approaching self-reflection is to write from the heart. What are you dealing with at the moment and how do you truly feel about it? Set a timer and just pour out any thoughts and feelings, and notice how it can be both therapeutic and eye opening. There really isn't a wrong way to approach this idea of self-reflection as long as it's approached with truthfulness (*satya*), discipline (*tapas*) and without judgement or criticism (*ahimsa*).

Self-reflection is about looking at the ways you react, your beliefs, thoughts and how you feel. Analyse how your reactions impact things and whether a different reaction may cause a more positive result.

I read a beautiful novel called *How Yoga Works* by Geshe Michael Roach and there's a poignant scene in the book about a bamboo pen. The yoga teacher asks her student what the object is and he responds that, of course, it is a pen. She proceeds to pass this 'pen' out of the window and give it to a cow who then eats it. The cow's reality is, this object is food. It's easy to think we all see the world in the same way, but our layers colour our vision. Having the ability to see things from multiple perspectives allows us to let go of categories and labels which can make us rigid. We need to be supple and adaptive, remember the concept of *sukha*, or ease. We need to stay curious and test the edges and layers that we have in place.

Self-study can help us connect to what actually matters and our true beliefs. It helps to set ourselves free from our created reality and the restraints we can make for ourselves. It invites us to tune in and pay attention, noticing when we are doing something because someone else wants us to, or even because our mind thinks that is what we should be doing. Pleasing the world is impossible; instead, start to learn how to truly please and trust yourself.

At some point in our lives many of us stop trusting the voice within and we turn outside for validation. We end up living life but not actually *living* our life. Make your own decisions from your core and to help you know what that is, journaling can help you sink down into a new level within yourself.

LET'S GO

Below are the starter questions to help you on your self-reflection journey. Remember that everything you need is inside of you. When you start tuning in and paying attention, you can work out what drives you, what's important in your life and what makes you happy.

Questions:

▸ What three things are you going to work on this week?

▸ What are five things you love about yourself?

▸ What are five things you love about someone else?

▸ What activities would you love to try but haven't made time for and why?

▸ Think about the last time you reacted in a way that you regretted. What made you react in that way? Can you think about how you can avoid this going forward?

▸ Write down one behavioural pattern that is not serving you and is causing suffering. What can you do differently? How does it feel to challenge this habit?

▸ Bring your mind to a situation where your view was clouded by beliefs and past experiences. What can you learn from this and do differently next time?

▸ What are your top priorities right now? Is there anything else you want to priotise?

▸ Reflect on a situation where you believed you were better or worse than others around you. Now think about something you could teach or learn from those people.

▸ Think back to the last time you heard someone saying bad words against you. What was your reaction? What could you do differently next time?

▸ Imagine you were told you only had three months left to live. What would you do differently? What would remain unchanged?

▸ Think back to the last time you went to a yoga class that was slightly different to usual. Notice the attachment you may have to your familiar practice and how moving at a different pace or style makes you feel.

▸ When was the last time you got so engrossed in a task that everything around you seemed to fade? Can you bring more of this into your life?

▸ What in your life are you unable to control and how does that make you feel? Is there anything you can do about it?

THE EGO AND THE *KLESHAS*

In the *Yoga Sūtras of Patañjali*, there are five obstacles or afflictions of the mind which hide our true self and they are known as the *kleshas*. They are thought to be the cause of negative reactions instead of positive ones, and are regarded as the source of all suffering. They are also thought to be buried deep inside our being, so it's helpful to know a bit about them when thinking about the idea of self-study. *Kleshas* can become stronger or weaker through behavioural patterns, and conscious action is key in weakening them (rather than unconscious reaction).

THE FIVE *KLESHAS* ARE:

▶ **AVIDYA** This is a lack of awareness, understanding or ignorance. This root *klesha* is at the core of the other *kleshas* which can only exist if *avidya* is present. When we have awareness, open-mindedness and see things clearly, we witness the truth and as a result there is less suffering.

▶ **ASMITA** This is egotism, or insecurity, and feeling more, or less, than you really are. The physical, emotional and mental aspects of the mind and body are mistaken for the true self. *Asmita* can be thought of as believing that our being is limited to things like our name, job title or age. The ego is like a lens showing us the world in a certain way, an interpretation of reality. It is important to have a healthy ego, not seeing yourself as worse or better than others, and being able to welcome feedback, not taking offence at criticism.

▶ **RAGA** This can be thought of as an attachment to the pleasurable parts of life. Although at first this may not seem like an issue, it can become a problem if we can't deal with not having the things we are used to. It's like going to a friend's, asking for a cup of tea but feeling frustrated or disappointed when the tea isn't just how we like it. Over time these annoyances can add up and have an impact on your life.

▶ **DVESA** The opposite to *raga*, this is the resistance to things we do not like. *Dvesa* is when this aversion changes how we act in a way that isn't helpful for us. No one enjoys unpleasant experiences – for example, going for a filling at the dentist. But avoiding and hiding from the pain of bad experience is stored in our bodies and mind. Each time a *dvesa* appears use it as an opportunity to study what your reaction wants to be and instead choose to consciously act. On your yoga mat, notice which poses you 'don't like' and notice how it is this resistance, not the pose itself, that is the actual cause of your suffering.

▶ **ABHINIVESA** This is attachment to life and fearing death. Accepting that death is unescapable can bring freedom. Use *abhinivesa* as a reminder to appreciate the present moment and live life to the full.

SELF-STUDY ON THE MAT

The idea of self-study flows onto the yoga mat. A person's physical practice and habits within it can reveal a lot about their life off the mat. When practising yoga we have to pay attention; the daily distractions of our phone, to-do lists, the news... they aren't there. It makes us aware of how we are breathing, moving and where the mind is going, and it shows us what we may need to work on.

We bring focus to the breath, which can make us realise how we haven't paid any attention to it recently. Tuning in and noticing what the breath looks like can help us understand how we are feeling. Maybe we are feeling stressed and anxious and the breath is stuck in the chest. Can we identify the root cause of this stress and anxiety and at the same time deepen the breath to bring our body some calm and restoration? And when you're practising, can you notice when you lose the breath, maybe moving too dynamically, and can you take a moment to come back to it and refocus?

Can you also unearth feelings of unnecessary tension – the belly, shoulders and jaw being classic examples? I have discussed previously the idea of effort and ease. Notice where you are holding tension that you don't need, and see if you can release it. Try to identify when this tension starts to creep in and why. Notice where you might be pushing yourself in your practice too much and instead can you find a modification that feels better for your body? Or take a moment to pause and breathe. When we keep checking in, we stay in touch with any emotions, feelings, thoughts and sensations taking place within our bodies.

With yoga we are trying to still the fluctuations of the mind, but it can feel impossible to find focus and quiet. Instead of thinking about clearing the mind, simply recognise and acknowledge the thoughts coming in and gently let them go. As you flow around the mat notice what thoughts come up; in longer holds I often tell my students to tune in and notice how their mind reacts, or where it wanders off to. Practising this over time you'll start to notice patterns, which in turn will make you aware of other aspects of yourself.

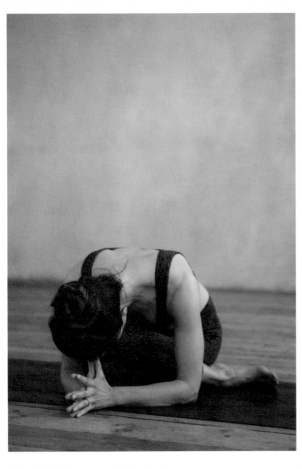

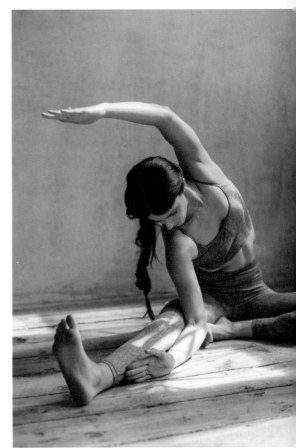

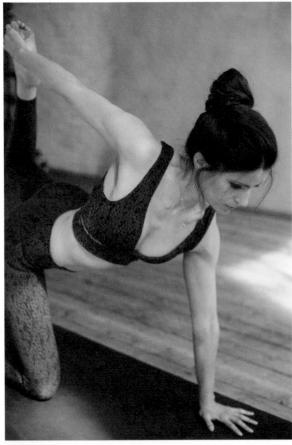

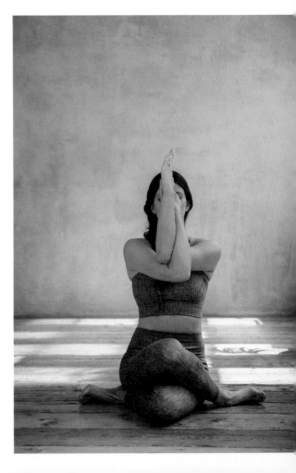

FIND
FULFILMENT
AND GROWTH

'HAPPINESS IS A STATE OF
INNER FULFILMENT.'

MATTHIEU RICARD

Life lessons sometimes come to us from unexpected places. One such experience in my life was when my grandmother passed away. We were close and I felt like a hole was left where she once shone. I longed to be reconnected to her. Then, about two months after she died, the people who bought her flat found her wedding ring, which she had lost years before. Incredibly they took the time to send it back to us with a little note, and that simple act of honesty and kindness from a stranger has had a lasting impact. I have since worn her ring every single day and it's a perpetual reminder both that she remains with me in happy memories, and of the good in people's hearts, even those you've never met. These feelings reflect two of the *yamas* (moral disciplines): *ahimsa* (non-violence or kindness) and *satya* (truthfulness). They show us that simple acts of kindness have the ability to transform the lives of both the giver and the receiver.

The *yamas* and *niyamas* are ethical principles intended to guide how we behave in a compassionate manner both towards others and towards ourselves. The *yamas* set out what you should avoid doing, which would be harmful to both you and others. The *niyamas* set out what you should do for the good of both you and others. They are the foundation for a meaningful and life-changing yoga path and over time will transform how you look at and approach life and your relationships. They will help you create transformation and happiness both inwardly and out in the world.

These principles can seem overwhelming at first, but they are the roots of our whole yoga practice. In this chapter I will help break their meanings down and show you how they can apply to your yoga practice (on the mat) and also to your life in general (off the mat), to help make sense of the world and your role in it.

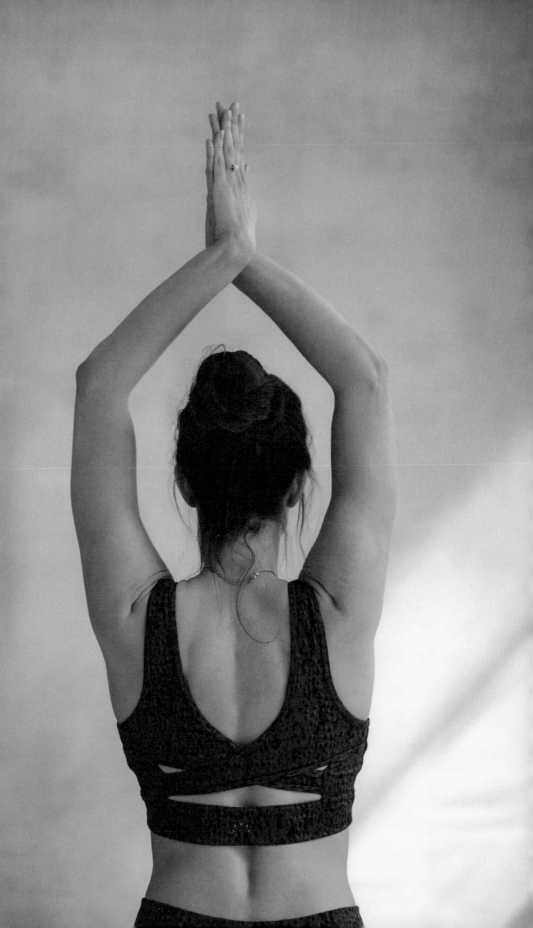

YAMAS

AHIMSA – non-violence in thought, word and deed

SATYA – truthfulness

ASTEYA – non-stealing

BRAHMACHARYA – celibacy or the 'right use of energy'

APARIGRAHA – non-possessiveness or non-attachment

Yamas can be thought of like an ethical backbone. They guide our behaviour so that we avoid actions that are harmful either to ourselves or to other people. We have an opportunity to practise their philosophy through any and every interaction with another living being. The way we treat others can reflect how we feel about life in general – especially as it relates to us. Take someone who is never happy or feeling content with life – the kind of person who thinks nothing is ever good enough. Sadly, they are often the ones who treat others the worst.

Remember two things: firstly, we *all* share the same divine inner light, we are no better or worse than one another, we are just all modelled by different experiences which shape us and affect the way we behave; secondly, remember that we can write the narrative and happiness is a choice. Bringing the concepts from this chapter into your daily life is going to have a *huge* impact on you and on others.

I think of the *yamas* as sharing the love of yoga. The more you practise them, the more they will benefit not only you but others too. With them you are planting positive seeds of change for others to follow so that they behave with a strong ethical backbone as well.

NIYAMAS

SAUCHA – cleanliness of the body, heart, mind and surroundings

SANTOSHA – contentment

TAPAS – discipline or to practise causing positive change

SVADHYAYA – study of the self and of sacred texts

ISHVARA PRANIDHANA – humility, faith, surrender to a higher being

These can be thought of as internal *yamas* as they bring attention to our body and surroundings. This links to the next chapter, in which we talk about self-care, because if we can't take care of ourselves, how can we expect to take care of others? And like the *yamas*, our behaviour has a huge impact on those around us. Whether you have children or simply think about family and friends, if we treat ourselves with care, respect, love and kindness we are setting the best example for them to follow. Like the *yamas*, the *niyamas* help us plant positive seeds of change for others to emulate.

As much as these classic descriptions of the *yamas* and *niyamas* sound great, the question is how can these work in practice and what do they really mean? Over the page is my take on each principle to help you consider how you can integrate them into your life.

There are lots of different views on what the *yamas* and *niyamas* mean and it's up to you to decide what they mean to you and how you want to put them into practice.

THE *YAMAS* IN PRACTICE

AHIMSA – NON-VIOLENCE

At the heart of yoga is love. *Ahimsa* doesn't just relate to violence and harm towards others but also to yourself and not just in the physical sense but in all senses. When we harm others, whether through thoughts, words or actions, we are also harming ourselves. And the opposite is true too.

With *ahimsa* we must practise non-discrimination, non-judgement and forgiveness. We are responsible for our own thoughts, words and actions and we can choose to demonstrate love and kindness.

All of the *yamas* and *niyamas* should be practised with *ahimsa* in mind.

Off the mat:

▶ Bring to mind someone that you don't paticularly like. Can you look at this person instead with feelings of love, compassion and kindness? Next time you see this person, notice if this changes how you feel.

▶ Non-violence towards others can also be about letting them go through their own challenges without trying to fix things for them, giving them the opportunity to learn from the situation. Notice if there is someone in your life that you're always trying to fix or save. Instead, be with them and give them the gift of listening and supporting them without taking charge of their life.

▶ *We* are responsible for, and have choice over, our thoughts, words and actions. If we surround ourselves with negativity, violence and unkindness, this is going to rub off on us. Consciously make a choice this week to reduce experiences that expose you to violence. This can include what you watch, where you shop (are you supporting ethical businesses?) and who you spend time with, among other things. Surround yourself instead with as much kindness and purity as possible and notice how this makes you feel.

On the mat:

▶ On the yoga mat can you honour and love your body and truly listen to whether you need any modifications to avoid harm?

SATYA – TRUTHFULNESS

Satya is present when our thoughts, words and actions are consistent and honest. It goes hand in hand with *ahimsa*, as clear and honest communication prevents harm. There is also a sense of transience in truth because of this marriage between *satya* and *ahimsa*. *Ahimsa* stops us from using the truth to hurt others – for example, when my daughter Amelie comes to me with a picture of her rainbow that in fact resembles a cookie, a softer approach to the truth is much more appropriate. Remember that words hold immense power and can cause happiness or grief (see pages 100–111).

Off the mat:

▶ Notice any tendency you have to gossip. Can you instead ask questions, have compassion and an open mind and seek out other sides of the story before judgement? Notice how this makes you feel in comparison to gossiping.

▶ Do you ever model yourself like play dough into a different shape for different people? Can you instead strive for 'realness'? Real isn't always liked and it can be scary and make us feel vulnerable – but if we live a life that isn't real in the hope of being nice and everyone liking us, it's just going to cause us suffering. There's pain in people not knowing the real you; in not being known.

On the mat:

▶ Notice where you may not be being truthful with yourself. Are you ignoring an area of your body where you are feeling particularly tight, or an area of pain? Can you modify your practice according to what your body needs, rather than what your mind thinks you need?

ASTEYA – NON-STEALING

Non-stealing can sound like a very obvious thing to avoid but it isn't just about taking something physical that doesn't belong to us. It can be about not stealing people's time or energy, not stealing people's opportunity to speak or share, not stealing too much from the earth and not moving in a way we are not ready for.

To help cultivate *asteya*, practise feeling contentment and satisfaction with the life you're living right here and now. Doing this means there is nothing you want to take; there is nothing more that you need.

Off the mat:

▶ How many times has someone told you a story and you're not fully present when listening to it? Maybe you were thinking about something different, about what you want to say in response, or even simply thinking, 'What can I say to make that person feel better?'. Can you try practising being completely present when listening? Give them the gift of your full attention, not stopping their flow and chance to unload. Don't make the story about you.

▶ Consider how much you're taking from the Earth – it could be food, clothes, space – and think about the necessity for these items and the impact on the planet you are leaving for your grandchildren, for your great-great-great grandchildren. Instead of wanting more 'things' can you take a moment to appreciate everything around you that brings joy and isn't typically 'owned' – nature, museums, or a rainbow when the rain meets the sun? Can you think of ways you can find your joy elsewhere without having to acquire more things?

On the mat:

▶ In your yoga practice, your focus should be on you, just you. Tune in and notice, are you trying to practise and look the same as an advanced yogi without having the right foundations? In itself this is a form of stealing, wanting more before it's your time to have it.

BRAHMACHARYA – 'RIGHT USE OF ENERGY'

Brahmacharya relates to conserving energy (traditionally sexual energy) so that you can channel it into better directions. It was even interpreted as celibacy or abstinence – striving for non-excess in our sexual desires and passion.

Although this can be thought of as the literal translation it also applies to life on and off the mat in different ways. Yoga teaches us moderation and balance, making sure that we're enjoying life but not becoming too attached or addicted to certain things. *Brahmacharya* is about spending energy where it's needed and recognising where it isn't. Cherish and respect all life energy. Although it can be renewed, energy isn't infinite and we need to make sure we're not pushing ourselves too much (or too little).

Off the mat:

▸ Think about where you're spending your energy. Can you think about the activities that fall into your days and notice whether you are finding the right balance and right use of your energy?

▸ Find the benefit in slowing down. What aspects of life are you overdoing – food, drink, partying, working,? Slow down and notice when something goes from being a pleasure to being too much.

On the mat:

▸ In your practice think about your use of energy. Are you pushing yourself to do a pose which felt good yesterday but isn't right for you today? We are forever changing and need to evolve to allow for this.

APARIGRAHA – NON-ATTACHMENT

Aparigraha is practising non-grasping and applies to material things, our bodies and our thoughts. It teaches us to take only what we need, to enjoy what we have, and to let go when the time is right.

On page 120 I discussed the ego, and the ego feeds on greed. As we accumulate more and more material things, money or whatever else it is, this all feeds our ego. However, when we look at life through a clear lens, we realise that we don't want this superficial existence; that happiness and contentment and everything we need is within us. Nothing stays the same: life is continually changing, so attachment and grasping on to life as it is now is the cause of suffering; it's not the change itself. Free yourself from a sense of 'clinging on' and in turn find freedom.

Off the mat:

▶ Look around your house and find something you haven't used for over six months. Ask yourself, why are you clinging on to it and can you not share it instead with others so that it can be loved like it was designed to be? Practise non-attachment.

▶ Think about how to reduce your footprint on this Earth in terms of what you buy. For example, do you truly need more clothes in your wardrobe?

▶ Take the concept of *aparigraha* into the conversations you have with others. Notice if you have the fluidity to listen to others or to believe someone else could have an opinion of value. *Aparigraha* stops us from believing we are a higher power and everyone else should be just listening to us.

On the mat:

▶ Practise yoga for the love of practising. Don't force things or push yourself to the limit – that *asana* that seems impossible in this moment will become accessible over time.

▶ Next time you go to a yoga class with a new teacher or style that you weren't expecting, try to drop all attachments and 'go with the flow'.

THE *NIYAMAS* IN PRACTICE

SAUCHA – CLEANLINESS

The first *niyama* means cleanliness or purity of the body, heart and mind. This applies to your entire life, from keeping the body clean, to the things you eat, your living space, even to your thoughts, words and actions. When our body and mind are clear, everything else in life becomes easier.

Off the mat:

▸ Find the messiest room in your house and clean it thoroughly putting everything away in its proper place. How does this affect your state of mind?

▸ Use *saucha* as a reminder to slow down, to be pure with each moment without hurrying through life in a frenzy. Notice how often you have the tendency to rush to the next thing in life, and instead see if you can slow down and truly pay attention to the present moment.

On the mat:

▸ Cleanliness of movement can be in terms of alignment but also relates to intention. Can you be mindful as you flow around the mat? Imagine that you are flowing through honey or treacle, paying attention to each transition and the moments in each pose. Bring your full awareness to each sensation and the breath.

▸ *Saucha* also invites purity with who we truly are. Recognise when you may not be allowing yourself to feel or think a certain way. Notice when you may be hiding from your true self.

SANTOSHA – CONTENTMENT

Santosha can be thought of as contentment or gratitude. It invites us to find gratitude for what we do have and not search for what we don't.

True happiness comes from feeling content with who we are and what we have at this moment. Not looking for anything else, allowing life to change from moment to moment, and having complete satisfaction and contentment within. It helps us to connect with the moments that matter and invites us to love life as is.

If you start practising this today and have the discipline to take a pause every day to recognise some of the good in your life, in two months you'll notice a big shift in your overall contentment.

Off the mat:

▶ Next time you find yourself in a queue or waiting for something you didn't expect to have to wait for, try to find joy in the moment – a way to enjoy this precious time of being still.

▶ *Santosha* is finding contentment with the sunny days and equally the rainy ones. Next time you're having a bad day or simply thinking, 'I'll be happier if…', can you find gratitude? It can be as simple as an inhale and exhale. A reminder that you are alive right here and now.

▶ Close your eyes and think of three things that you're grateful for right now.

On the mat:

▶ Find joy and contentment in each moment, each pause, each breath.

The last three *niyamas* – *tapas*, *svadhyaya* and *ishvara pranidhana* – are defined as *kriya* yoga. When used together, these three tools are powerful for learning and growth and can help bring inner change. Author Leslie Kaminoff once pointed out that these three tools are just like the famous Serenity Prayer. *Ishvara pranidhana* grants us the serenity to accept the things we cannot change. *Tapas*, fire and dedication in practice, grants us the courage to change the things we can. *Svadhyaya* or 'self-study', gives us the wisdom to know the difference between what we can and cannot change.

TAPAS – DISCIPLINE

With *tapas* we practise causing positive change. *Tapas* means 'heat' and can be translated as catharsis, transformation or burning enthusiasm and self-improvement. It means having the courage to change the things that you can, and the dedication and fire to take action towards a goal. *Tapas* keeps our mind, body and breath moving and free from stagnation.

Discipline can be hard. We've discussed how starting an *asana* practice is extremely difficult but the more you practise the more transformation you see. The same can be seen from breaking free of habits that don't serve you. Yoga helps us to transform both internally and externally and it's a lifelong journey.

Off the mat:

▸ To put *tapas* in motion, set an intention to commit to positive change in your life and write down exactly what it is that you want to do. Start with small changes and over time add in more and more, fanning the flames of tapas so that your fire burns brighter.

▸ *Tapas* can be both transformative and destructive. Think about the things in your life you are trying to change. Are there some in fact that don't need changing?

On the mat:

▸ When you practise try pushing yourself a little bit more than you have before (of course without risking injury) and feel the response this has on your body, on your muscles. For example, hold chair pose for that extra few breaths. Feel the heat of *tapas* and notice how this makes you feel.

SVADHYAYA – SELF-STUDY

In the previous chapter I spoke about self-study in respect of tuning inwards and reflecting deeply on your practice, thoughts, beliefs and behaviour. Yoga on and off the mat allows you to get to know yourself better, to get to know your body as you move, and to get to know how your mind works in both chaos and stillness.

Svadhyaya isn't just about analysing our emotions, thoughts and our mind but analysing anything that elevates our mind and reminds us of our true self. It is therefore also the study of sacred texts (for example the *Yoga Sūtras of Patañjali*, *The Bhagavad Gita* and *The Hatha Yoga Pradipika*), and not in the way of inhaling as many texts as possible but truly *reading* them and *understanding* them.

Traditionally *svadhyaya* also meant learning and repeating a purifying mantra chosen for you by your teacher. Repeating the mantra is a way to anchor the mind to one thought thus drawing awareness inward, quietening the outward aspects of the mind. See page 96 for a mantra meditation technique you can use to help with self-study.

Off the mat:

▶ If you haven't started already, begin to journal. For much more detail on this, turn to pages 116–119, but at the end of each day reflect on something that didn't quite go as planned and ask yourself why this happened and how tomorrow can be a new day.

▶ Do you have a book that you pick up again and again and each time learn something different from it? It's like it speaks to you at that moment and opens your eyes in a different way each time. Identify a book that you want to read (maybe one you've already read) and immerse yourself in it. Learn from it and put into practice what you have learnt, not just rushing on to the next book.

▶ Identify a time when you reacted in a way that you were not proud of. See if you can trace your reaction to a belief you are either consciously or unconsciously holding. Think about what you would have liked to have done instead and learn from this.

On the mat:

▶ Study the way you move. Discover parts of the body that you aren't usually aware of (the sensations along the back of your arms or the side of your torso, for example), discover how your practice feels when you change the way you breathe, and observe the mind and how it loves to wander when you come into *savasana* but focuses when you practise plank.

ISHVARA PRANIDHANA − SURRENDER

The final *niyama* invites us to surrender to something higher than ourselves and cultivate a path of non-resistance. If you are religious this may be easy for you to understand, as your connection to a higher power may be your god. But even if you aren't religious, you can think of the higher power as simply the sanctity of life. We are all share the same inner light, wrapped inside layers that are always changing. We need faith to help rid us of the fear of the unknown, of change. We need faith in a higher power to accept that whatever happens is meant to happen, even if it doesn't match what we expect. It helps us to release our attachments.

Ishvara pranidhana is said to lead to *samadhi*. *Samadhi* means enlightenment or bliss, and this is only attainable when we dedicate everything in life to a higher power and remove all attachments. I believe that this doesn't mean we only need to dedicate everything to a god (if you believe in a god) but also to humanity. Dedicate your life to the benefit of humanity and be mindful in everything you do.

Off the mat:

▶ Notice the tendency to label something as a bad day if things don't go the way you planned. Can you instead think of this change of plan as what was meant to happen, find fluidity and lose the attachment to the way that you wanted it to happen?

▶ There's a beautiful quote by the spiritual leader Swami Sivanandaji that says, *'Convert every work into yoga with the magic wand of right attitude.'* So think about giving everything a yogic touch. Next time you want to slam a door, close it gently, with love – remember that door has history, such as the tree it came from, the many different people it took to make the wood into the door and to place it in your house. Show all humanity love.

▶ If you find yourself worrying about something ask yourself if you can change it, or if you can't. If you can change it, do something; if you can't, there's no reason to worry about it. Let go of what you can't change, and allow yourself to grow more and live life fully.

On the mat:

▶ Come to each practice with a heart of devotion. Devote your practice to someone or something. Start with an offering, maybe lighting a candle or burning incense. Move around your mat with the intention of surrender and explore any resistance.

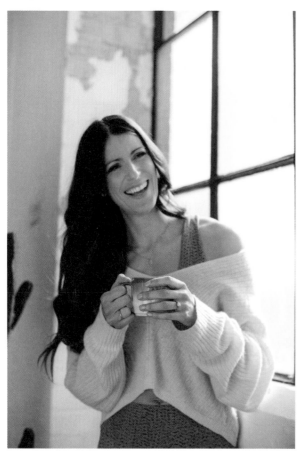
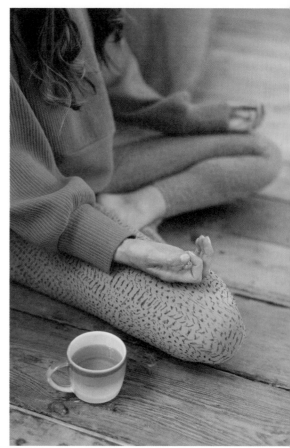
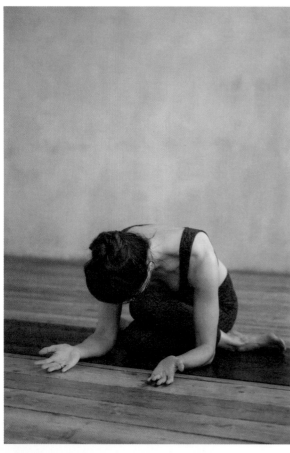
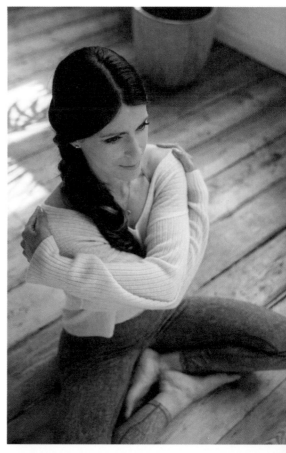

SELF-CARE
AND
CONNECTION

'TALK TO YOURSELF LIKE YOU
WOULD TO SOMEONE YOU LOVE.'

BRENÉ BROWN

When I worked in finance as an actuary I could go months working all hours under the sun, pushing myself to do more, more, more and accepting projects I should have said no to. I didn't listen out for the messages that suggested my body needed rest until it was too late. It was a common occurrence that whenever I did take time off to have a break, I would end up sick – usually manifesting itself as tonsillitis – which is really not what you want on a two-week holiday. I didn't listen, I didn't tune in and I didn't stop. If I had done, I would have been happier and also better at my job.

I felt a shift in my life when I took a moment to really define what success meant to me. I had grown up with the view that success was a big family, lots of friends, my own house and a job that paid well. But what are all of these things if you aren't happy? I realised that for me (and for you it could be completely different) success was feeling happy, content and like I had purpose. There's no doubt that had I discovered yoga earlier I would have been better at my old job, because not only has yoga taught me the importance of self-care and tuning inwards, but it has helped me handle stress better, improved my focus and concentration, and has had a huge impact on my self-esteem. Instead of hustling through my days I could have taken a step back to connect with what was important. This point I am making goes far beyond what job we have and applies to the whole of our lives. We need connection and we need to truly love ourselves. We *can* find happiness, we can *choose* happiness.

Before reading the rest of this chapter I invite you to take a pause and jot down what success means to you. No judgement, you don't need to show anyone. But once you have this idea clear in your mind, think about what you do day to day and notice where you can make changes to align with your view of success and to create more happiness in your life. So as an example, with my old job I would have placed boundaries around my working hours. These would have, of course, been flexible because at times things just need to be done, but working crazy-hour weeks regularly out of choice wasn't beneficial to anyone.

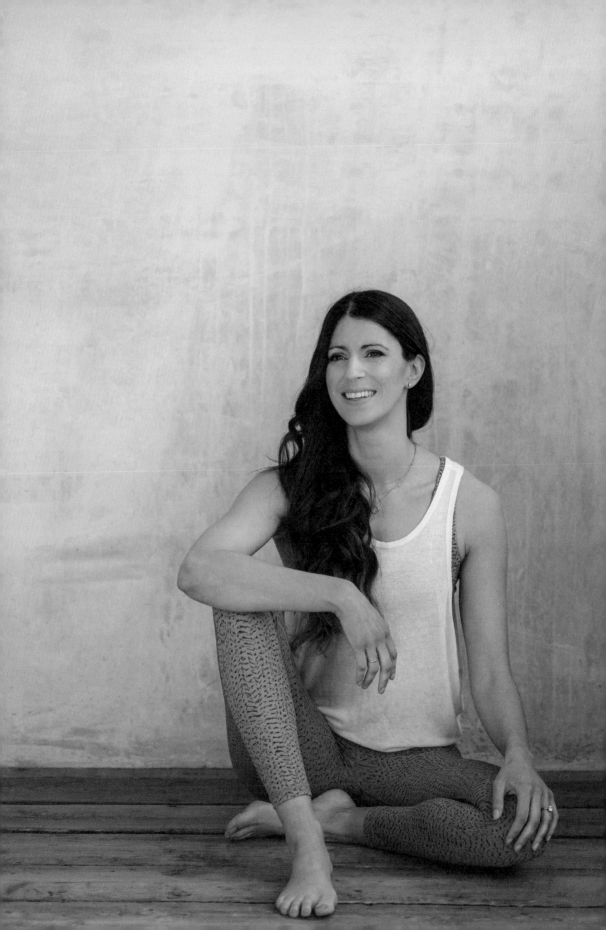

HAPPINESS IS A CHOICE

When my son was two, I took him out for a purposeful walk in the rain for the first time. He was blown away by everything: the umbrella, the puddles, the sounds, the feeling of the water on his skin. He devoured everything about the moment and it was beautiful to watch. It made me realise how much of life's simple pleasures are easy to miss, and how the things we perceive as negative can be flipped on their heads – like getting rained on. Children are the masters of living in the present, finding happiness in the smallest of things, and in that moment he taught me so much about reconnecting with my inner child and it felt immense. I now look forward to rainy days as I bundle the kids up into rain suits and wellies and we splash around getting muddy beyond belief. These small pleasures, they matter. Cling on to these small moments as years down the line you'll look back and see how big they really were.

Happiness being a choice can be hard to hear if you are struggling. I have suffered with severe depression in the past and know that just choosing to be happy wouldn't have been a magic fix or even an option at the time. There are no magic quick-fixes, and if you are struggling with depression or anxiety that is impacting your life please speak to a trusted health professional for help. The feeling of being alone can be overwhelming and horrible and I know that feeling well. Reach out and ask for help; it was the best thing I ever did.

What I learnt through the process of recovery is that small steps lead to big changes. The tools that I have shared throughout this book *do* help. Day one of a gratitude practice probably won't give you an explosion of happiness but on day 100 you will realise the significant impact it has had on how you view life, in what you view as important, and in your happiness levels. Day one of a meditation practice is probably going to feel extremely difficult, maybe even impossible. By day 100 you are going to be looking forward to it – to a moment of calm between the chaos. All of these things add up and over time they have a immense impact on how much you can find connection in your life and they can make you realise the beauty in life. These tools will build up your resilience for the bumps (or even craters) along your road.

We have to take part in the creation of our own happiness every single day. I've spoken earlier about practising mindfulness in everyday life (see pages 84–87). Can you find beauty in what you may have previously seen to be boring or even frustrating? When you find yourself waiting in a queue you didn't foresee, can you find joy in the moment and embrace this time to just be and watch the people around you? Notice how connected they are in themselves. Are they looking calm and happy, or are they rushing around with their face in a screen? I find when I do this it's a reality check on how I want to live life. I want to be the person paying attention to people and what's right in front of them.

WHAT IS SELF-CARE?

It took me a long time to grasp self-care. Many of us, not least parents, either put others first or forget entirely to allow ourselves to do things just for us – even if that's just eating well or listening to music after the kids have gone to bed. The fact is, if you aren't good to yourself, you stand less of a chance of being strong for others. It isn't about being selfish – it's about remembering that you, too, deserve to have a fulfilling, nourishing life and that all the things you value like kindness, gratitude and forgiveness, will actually be easier to give if you're happy and content in yourself. Self-care is neither optional nor selfish, it is *necessary*.

Self-care is about identifying what drives your contentment, joy, fulfilment and positive mental health, and then allowing yourself to actually do these things. About 99 times out of 100, what we think are barriers are put there by ourselves. How many times have you denied yourself doing something you love or kept working past exhaustion for fear of losing control of what's going on around you? How often do you feel like you 'should' be taking care of mundane things like cleaning the kitchen or doing laundry rather than stopping to feel the sun on your face or other such simple joys? By giving yourself value, and believing you deserve the care and respect you would show others, your strength will grow and you will begin to understand the difference between selfishness and self-fulfilment.

Self-care can look very different from day to day; it's a constant dialogue to check in with yourself. It isn't the idea that we need something to 'show' for our non-working hours. It is not a one-size-fits-all, and it doesn't need to be done in the 'right' way. It requires intention and the belief that it's worth our focus.

Yoga has taught me to remember I am human and to use self-care not just as a nice thing to do in the moment, but cumulatively as preventative medicine. Leaving the laundry for one day won't hurt you, but missing out on the experiences you love and value will. It's exactly the message I want to give to my children, because if they see me taking care of and valuing myself, they will do the same too.

SELF-CARE INSPIRATION

What do you love doing so much that you get completely immersed in it and lose all awareness of time? For me it's being in my yoga practice, reading and being outside in nature. Start to prioritise activities that have this joyful effect and notice how they add richness, fulfilment and fun to your life.

Here is some self-care inspiration, things that I love, that bring me delight and make me feel extremely connected. If these don't resonate with you, that's okay; ask yourself what you really want to do and just go for it.

▶ So much of our life is surrounded by technology, it's good to step away from digital interaction for part of our day to allow ourselves us to focus on real-life social interactions without distraction. Spending too much time behind screen can impact our sleep (as it suppresses the body's release of melatonin) and can make us feel less present and connected. Pick one happy activity that you *love* that isn't related to technology, whether it's reading, drawing, baking, playing a musical instrument, getting outside, whatever. Notice how you get lost in the moment.

▶ Nourish yourself well. As simple as this sounds, notice when you are hungry or when you need hydrating – it's easy to forget all this, especially when you're looking after others. At least three times this week have lunch without distraction. Even if it is simply putting your phone in another room, take time to just 'be' and mindfully appreciate the food you're nourishing your body with. Be conscious of the food that you put in your body but do allow yourself your favourite treats, too! Don't beat yourself up for a day involving too much chocolate; life is about balance. Listening to your body's needs is key.

▶ Practise morning mindfulness and connection. Instead of reaching for your phone or the TV remote first thing, take a moment to be still and meditate or journal, perhaps as you have a cup of tea and breakfast. Looking at your phone can be overloading and overwhelming and can increase stress and anxiety levels, giving you no time and space to start your day calmly. Instead of proactively starting the day focusing on your own goals, you're setting yourself up to react to other people's issues. Not only that, but you are primed for distraction for the rest of the day.

▶ Nourish yourself with nature. The tiniest patch of green will do. Turn off your phone and notice the sounds, the smells, the colours. Drink it all in. Research has shown that people who spend time in nature are healthier both physically and mentally. Nature is the antidote to today's busy and stressful world and provides an inexplicable sense of tranquil awareness.

▶ Consider animal therapy. Head to your nearest farm, zoo or wildlife centre and spend time noticing the different animals, the similarities and the noises they make, the things they do... Simply notice and connect. You can even observe the other people!

YOGA AND SELF-CARE

Yoga is the ultimate teacher of self-care. Throughout this book there has been a consistent message of 'tuning in' and finding connection. Through practising *asana* we are made more aware of how our body feels, our emotions and our mind. This means we are more likely to practise self-care and listen to what we need, when we need it; to know when we need to slow down and restore, and equally to know when we need to channel our energy into work, movement or creativity.

So many of the yogic principles will help guide your understanding of self-care:

AHIMSA: can be thought of as kindness towards yourself as much as towards other people;

SATYA: living your truth, saying no when no is needed and making time to nourish your body and mind;

ASTEYA: non-stealing, not letting life run away from you, not stealing your chance to live a full and happy life;

BRAHMACHARYA: the right use of energy, taking time to reset, breathe and look at your bucket of energy and know that this is a necessary part of life;

SAUCHA: purity or cleanliness, making the time to look after yourself, your body, your mind and your home.

Our yoga practice also teaches us perspective and the wisdom that around us is a larger world, and that our daily stresses may not be as big a deal as they initially seem. Life is magical and beautiful, and when we are kinder and gentler with ourselves we can see this beauty so much more, and we give back so much more to others too. Don't feel guilty for slowing down, saying no or putting your mental wellbeing first. As I said at the start of this book, you may have heard the phrase 'you can't pour from an empty cup'. Instead of just hearing it, truly *believe it*.

Good health requires you to take care of yourself and will help you drive the energy you desire out into the world. When we learn how to take care of ourselves, to value ourselves and believe we are worthy of self-care, it creates a ripple of positivity through our lives and into others.

Self-care doesn't have to be hot baths and stepping on your yoga mat. It can be reading, writing, dancing, meditation, painting; what it looks like doesn't matter, but you owe it to yourself to make it a daily priority. Make time to do the things in life that cause you joy, and in turn you'll find yourself more connected to your life. I challenge you to set aside at least 30 minutes each day for any self-care ritual of your choice. That's only 2 per cent of your day. Use it how you want to use it; make it count.

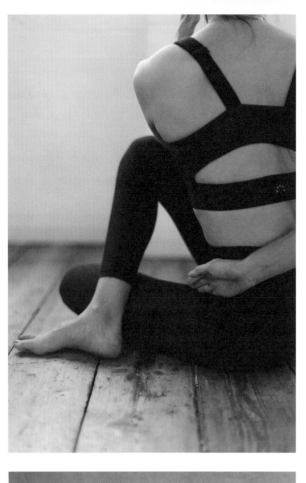

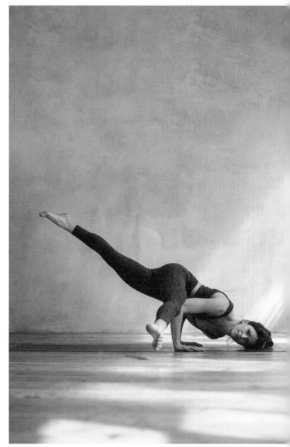

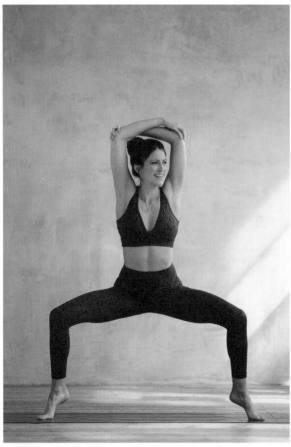

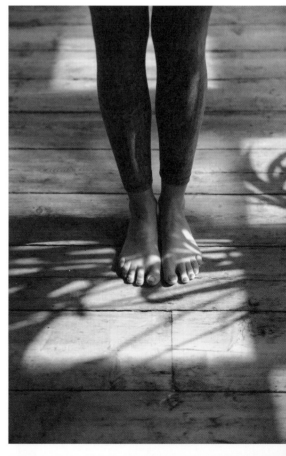

FINAL
THOUGHTS

'YOGA DOES NOT JUST CHANGE
THE WAY WE SEE THINGS,
IT TRANSFORMS THE
PERSON WHO SEES.'

B.K.S. IYENGAR

The final step in Patañjali's eight limbs of yoga is *samadhi*. It is the most complex of all the yogic concepts and is often defined as 'bliss', 'liberation' or 'enlightenment'. It is considered the highest state of consciousness, when you are in union and oneness with the Universe. When you have journeyed through the first seven limbs – finding compassion towards others (the *yamas*), taking care of yourself (the *niyamas*), moving (*asana*), breathing (*pranayama*), removing external stimuli (*pratyahara*), finding focus (*dharana*) and meditation (*dhyana*) – you are preparing for *samadhi*. Even the great yoga scholar B.K.S Iyengar observed: 'Nobody can say "I am in *samadhi*." One cannot talk or communicate. *Samadhi* is an experience where the existence of "I" disappears. Explanations can come only through the presence of "I", so *samadhi* cannot be explained.'

Travelling towards this state doesn't need you to move to an ashram. *Samadhi* isn't floating away on cloud nine; it's the act of recognising the life surrounding us and seeing this life equally, without judgement, without the mind disturbing us and without our experience being conditioned by external factors. It's about recognising the light within you, within others and everything surrounding you. We are all one with the Universe: nature, animals, people you love, and even people you don't like. We are all part of a continuum.

Every single moment in your life is an opportunity to practise the yoga journey towards *samadhi*. I invite you to find connection, awareness, ground yourself right here in the present moment, observe your relationship with others and yourself and to quieten all the noise. The path to balance requires listening, because it isn't always in the 'doing' –it can be about the 'undoing' too. If there is one takeaway I hope you find in this book, it is that every small step you take towards *samadhi* will help you to be increasingly more resilient, more compassionate and more joyful, no matter what life throws at you.

There is no rush. The healing power of yoga takes time, patience and practice. But the more you integrate yoga's teachings into your life on and off the mat, the more progress you will see. Remember the path is going to have highs and lows and each step is a step forwards – even when you fail, fail forwards. Learn from your mistakes and use them as an opportunity to grow. We are human, we all make mistakes. There is no 'perfect practice', or in fact you could look at every practice as perfect, giving us exactly what we need at that point in time. Follow the path, use the tools shared throughout this book and in time, happiness and contentment will become a natural part of your life.

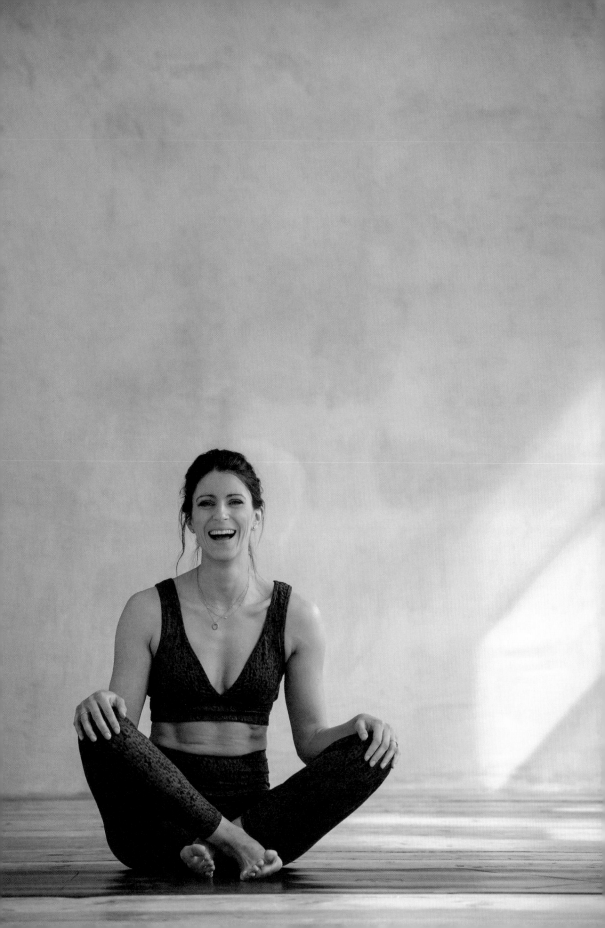

APPENDIX OF POSTURES

———

'AND I SAID TO MY BODY
SOFTLY, "I WANT TO BE YOUR
FRIEND". IT TOOK A LONG
BREATH AND REPLIED, "I HAVE
BEEN WAITING MY WHOLE
LIFE FOR THIS".'

NAYYIRAH WAHEED

BUTTERFLY POSE
(BADDHA KONASANA)

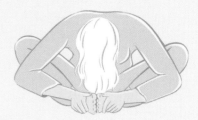

▶ From a seated position, bring the soles of your feet together letting the thighs gently open. Draw your feet in as close to your body as is comfortable (avoiding any pain in the knees).

▶ Gently interlace the fingers around the feet.

▶ Inhale and find length through the spine, exhale keeping the spine neutral and hinge forward from the hips as far as comfortable.

▶ Hold for 5 slow breaths, then gently inhale back up to centre and release.

▶ If hinging forwards feels too intense, stay upright. You can even use blocks or blankets under the thighs for added support.

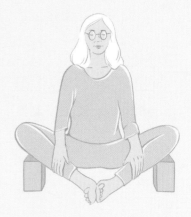

RECLINED BUTTERFLY POSE
(SUPTA BADDHA KONASANA)

▸ Lying on your back, bring the soles of the feet together letting the thighs gently open. Draw your feet in as close to your body as is comfortable (avoiding any pain in the knees).

▸ Place a blanket or blocks under the knees for support. Use blankets, pillows or bolsters behind the back, head and arms for ultimate relaxation.

▸ Stay for as long as needed, breathing mindfully.

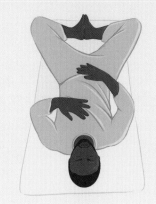

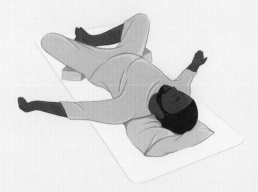

BRIDGE POSE
(*SETU BANDHASANA*)

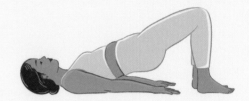

▸ Lie on your back with the knees bent, feet flat and hands by your side. Feet are hip width apart, toes pointing forward and heels about a hand's distance from the buttocks.

▸ Exhale and press into both feet lifting the hips off the floor, lengthening through the tailbone keeping the spine neutral and glutes engaged.

▸ Lengthen the back of the neck by gently nodding the chin down and hold for 5 breaths.

▸ Inhale and release the hips back towards the floor.

SUPPORTED BRIDGE POSE

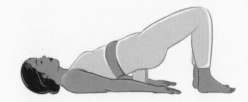

▸ Placing a block underneath the sacrum can be a really nice restorative version of this posture.

CAT AND COW
(*MARJARIASANA AND BITILASANA*)

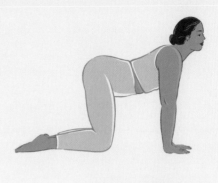

▶ Start on all fours, wrists directly under shoulders, knees directly under hips.

▶ Inhale into cow pose lifting the tailbone and arching the spine, having a sensation of pulling the hands backwards to help open the chest. Gaze forwards, keeping the neck long.

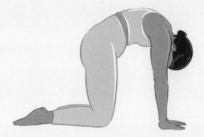

▶ Exhale into cat pose drawing the tailbone down and rounding the back, relaxing the head, drawing navel to spine and pushing the ground away to pull the shoulder blades away from the spine.

▶ Continue moving through cow and cat for 5 full breaths.

CHAIR POSE
(*UTKATASANA*)

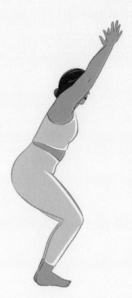

▸ Stand at the top of the mat, toes together, heels slightly apart.

▸ Inhale, raising the arms overhead (palms facing each other), lengthening the spine and bending the knees. Squeeze the knees together feeling the thighs and glutes fully engage avoiding any pain in the knees.

▸ If comfortable, gaze up between the hands, and keep the chest lifted and spine neutral, drawing the ribs in to avoid them flaring. Alternatively, keep the gaze forward.

▸ Hold the posture for 5 slow breaths.

▸ Option to modify by having the feet hip width apart.

CHILD'S POSE
(BALASANA)

▶ Kneel on the mat with the big toes together and the knees about hip width apart.

▶ Exhale and lay your torso down between the thighs keeping the spine long.

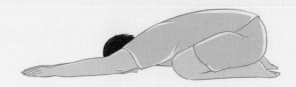

▶ Stretch the arms forwards feeling a stretch from the tailbone out through the fingertips.

▶ Alternatively, you can bring the knees together and/or bring the arms back and place the hands on the floor alongside the torso with the palms up, releasing the fronts of the shoulders toward the floor.

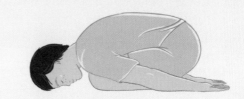

▶ Rest here for 5 slow breaths or longer if required.

▶ To make this pose really restorative, place a pillow between the thighs and melt the torso over it.

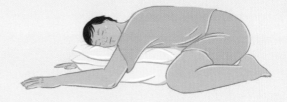

COBRA POSE
(*BHUJANGASANA*)

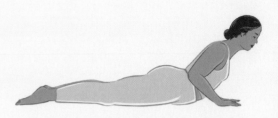

▸ Starting by lying on your belly, gently push
down through the tops of the feet and the pubic
bone, engaging through the glutes.

▸ Bring the hands underneath the shoulders
and as you inhale have the sensation of the
hands pulling backwards (without them
actually moving) to help lengthen the spine
and open the heart. Keep the neck long and
gaze slightly forward.

▸ Avoid pushing down through the floor and
use the muscles of the back instead drawing
the shoulder blades back and down. Engage
the glutes to help keep the pelvis neutral.

▸ Hold for 5 slow breaths and then exhale and
gently release.

DOLPHIN POSE
(ARDHA PINCHA MAYURASANA)

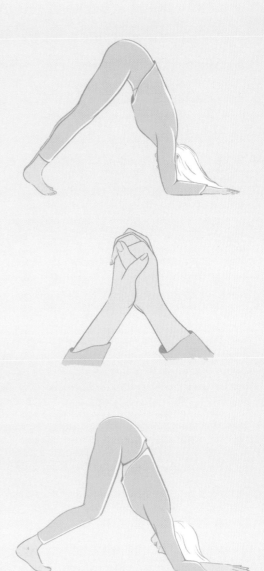

▸ Starting on hands and knees, lower the forearms and palms to the floor shoulder distance apart. If this feels too intense you can clasp the hands together (making a triangle shape with the arms).

▸ Release the head and push down firmly through the forearms drawing the shoulder blades away from your spine.

▸ Exhale and curl the toes under, lifting the knees away from the floor and the hips up.

▸ Lift the sitting bones up as you keep the spine long, drawing the heels down (if they don't touch the floor that's okay) and keeping as much of a bend in the knees as needed to keep the spine neutral.

▸ Draw the front ribs in towards the back body and hold the head between the upper arms, keeping the neck long.

▸ Hold for 5 breaths then exhale and slowly release.

DOWNWARD-FACING DOG POSE
(*ADHO MUKHA SVANASANA*)

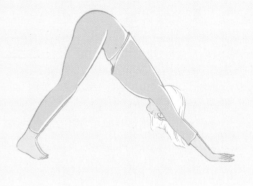

▶ Start on hands and knees with the hands shoulder distance and knees hip distance apart.

▶ Spread the fingers, middle finger facing straight ahead and press firmly into the mat through the whole hand. Have a sensation of 'dialing' the hands in opposite directions (like screwing jam jar lids) without the hands actually moving. This broadens and stabilises the shoulders.

▶ Exhale, curling the toes under and lifting the hips back and up reaching the sitting bones towards the ceiling, keeping the spine neutral. Keep the long spine as you start to slowly straighten the legs, avoiding any rounding in the lower back. Draw the heels towards the mat but don't worry if they don't reach. Keep the legs active by rotating the inner thighs inwards and firming the outer thighs.

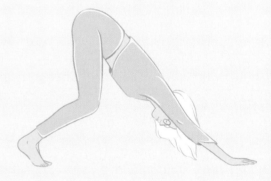

▶ Draw the front ribs in towards the back body.

▶ Keep the neck long, between the arms and hold for 5 breaths, then exhale and slowly release.

▶ Option to modify by bending the knees as much as you need to keep the spine long.

HALF-MOON POSE
(ARDHA CHANDRASANA)

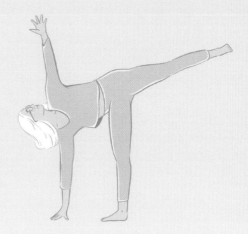

▶ Starting in warrior II (see page 178) with the right foot forward, inhale and slowly hinge the right side of the body forward over the right leg bringing the right hand towards the floor or onto a block in front of the right foot. As you shift the weight forward lift the left leg away from the mat, foot flexed or pointed.

▶ Roll the left hip back opening your body to the left, stacking the hips.

▶ Roll the left shoulder open to stack it over the right shoulder and either keep the left hand on the hip or extend the left arm straight up to the ceiling. Gaze either down at the ground or up at the hand.

▶ Hold for 5 slow breaths.

▶ Exhale and slowly return to warrior II using your core to help control the movement.

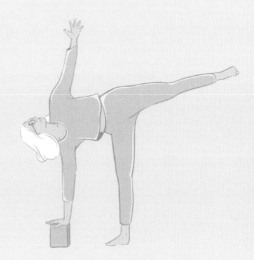

HAPPY BABY POSE
(*ANANDA BALASANA*)

▸ Lying on your back, bend the knees kicking the feet up towards the ceiling.

▸ Take hold of the outer edges of the feet, or the shins or thighs if preferred. Gently press the sacrum into the floor

▸ Take 5 slow breaths, maybe finding a gentle rocking sensation from side to side.

▸ A nice modification can be to do one side at a time.

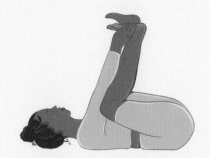

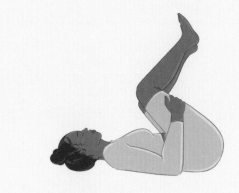

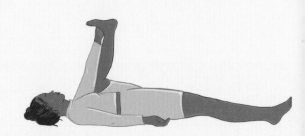

LAY DOWN KNEE ROCKS

► Lying on your back, bend your knees and bring the soles of the feet flat on the floor.

► Exhale and gently rock the knees over to the right keeping the hips down, and inhale back to centre.

► Repeat on the left then do 5–10 repetitions each side.

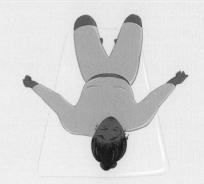

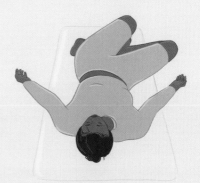

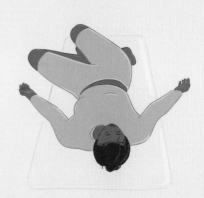

LEGS UP THE WALL POSE
(*VIPARITA KARANI*)

▶ Lying on a mat, bring the hips to the wall, with the upper body flat and sitting bones as close to the wall as is comfortable.

▶ Gently raise the legs straight up, resting them against the wall.

▶ Option to place a pillow or blanket under your sacrum to ease any discomfort in the lower back and help to hinge at the hips.

▶ If you have time, stay here for 5–15 minutes (or longer).

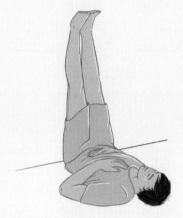

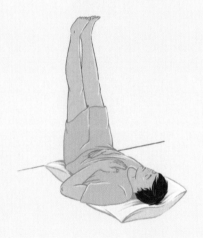

LIZARD POSE
(*UTTHAN PRISTHASANA*)

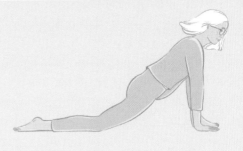

- From downward-facing dog pose (see page 160), exhale and step the right foot forward to the outside of the right hand (use your hand to help you if required) then come down onto the left knee. The further the knee is from the hands, the more intense the stretch in the hip flexor and quadricep (front of the thigh).

- Inhale as you find the sensation of pulling back in space with the hands (without moving them) to keep the spine long and the chest open.

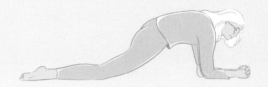

- Option to deepen the pose by either tucking the toes and lifting the back knee or coming down onto the forearms (ensuring that the spine stays long).

- Hold for 5 slow breaths.

- On the next exhale slowly release and repeat on the left side.

LOW LUNGE POSE
(ANJANEYASANA)

▸ From downward-facing dog pose (see page 160), exhale and step the right foot forward between the hands (use your hand to help you if required) coming down onto the left knee. Stack your right knee over your right ankle and the left hip over your left knee and engaging the glute to help open the front of the hip.

▸ Inhale and reach the fingers high to the sky, lengthening through the side body, drawing the ribs in to avoid them flaring.

▸ Hold for 5 breaths then repeat on the other side.

▸ Option to step the right foot forward further to focus the stretch on the front of the thigh, keeping the pelvis in a neutral position.

▸ Option to turn this into a backbend keeping the glutes strong and lifting the chest upwards gently opening through the upper spine.

▸ Place a blanket or cushion under the back knee if needed.

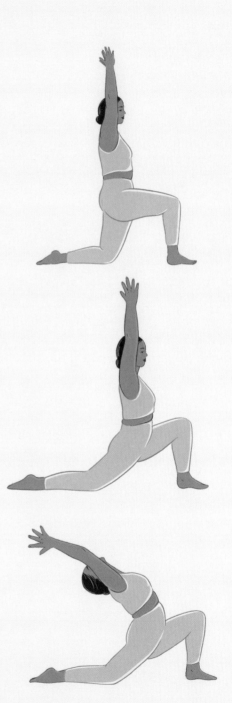

PLANK POSE
(PHALAKASANA)

▸ Come on to your hands and knees with the wrists under the shoulders.

▸ Step the feet back, tucking the toes and lifting the knees from the floor. The legs and glutes should be engaged.

▸ Bring the hips in line with the shoulders and keep a neutral spine with the neck long and gaze slightly forward. Avoid the lower back overarching or head dropping and draw the ribs in.

▸ Keep the arms strong and have a sensation of 'dialing' the hands in opposite directions (like screwing jam jar lids) and set the shoulder blades into a neutral position.

▸ Hold for 5 breaths then release.

▸ Option to modify this pose by dropping the knees – the closer the knees to the hands the less intense.

▸ Option to come onto the forearms with the knees down or lifted.

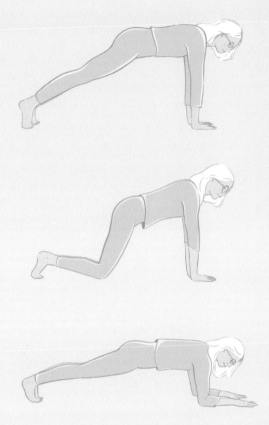

RESTORATIVE FISH POSE (*MATSYASANA*)

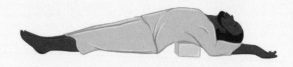

▶ Place a pillow or block parallel to the short edge of your mat about a foot and a half away from the back of the mat.

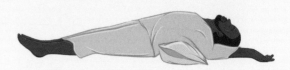

▶ Option to place another pillow or block for your head at the back of the mat. Gently lie back over the prop(s) bringing the bottom edge just below the tips of the shoulder blades and the other under your head (if desired).

▶ Melt the body over the prop(s) and place the arms to the side or overhead – whatever is most comfortable. Stay for 1–2 minutes or more. When exiting the pose gently roll to one side and remove the prop(s).

▶ Option to clasp the hands behind the head, opening the shoulders as much is comfortable. You can even take a gentle side to side movement with the upper back.

SAVASANA
(CORPSE POSE)

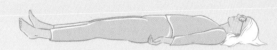

- Start by lying on your back with the feet mat distance apart and let the feet drop open. If there is any pain in the lower back, bend the knees, bringing the feet flat on the floor and letting the knees drop in towards each other.

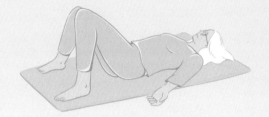

- Lay the arms by your sides away from the body, turning the palms to face the ceiling and letting the fingers curl in naturally. Relax the shoulder blades evenly on the mat and lengthen through the back of the neck.

- Close the eyes and allow the whole body to become soft and heavy, melting into the floor.

- Stay here for 5 deep breaths or as long as desired.

SEATED POSTURES
(*SUKHASANA*)

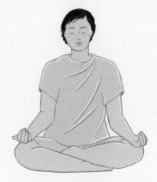

▸ Come onto the floor, crossing one leg in front of the other.

▸ Feel the sitting bones underneath you rooting down and find length in the spine.

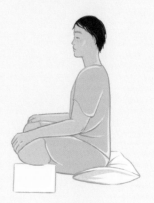

▸ If this is uncomfortable (as it is for many!) you can do these seated postures on a block or pillow to allow gradual release of the hips and help you find length in the spine. Option to also place pillows under the thighs.

▸ From this position you can roll the shoulders or gently move the head from side to side, up and down, moving mindfully with the breath.

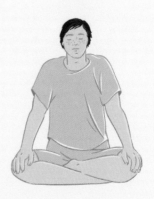

SEATED CAT AND COW

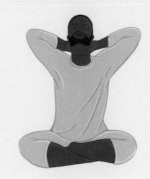

▶ From a seated position, interlace the fingers behind the head.

▶ Inhale as you open the elbows and chest, breathing up and lifting through the chest bringing a gentle bend into the upper spine.

▶ Exhale and start to round through the back bringing elbow to elbow as you draw navel to spine, round the back and tuck the chin.

▶ Repeat 5 times.

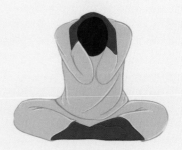

SEATED NECK STRETCH

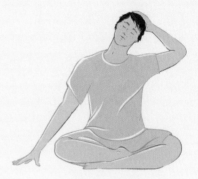

▶ From a seated position, gently rest the right fingertips on the ground beside the right hip.

▶ Take a breath in as you bring the left hand to the crown of the head, and as you breathe out slowly bring the left ear towards the left shoulder using the hand as a gentle guide.

▶ Take 5 breaths here and then inhale, release and repeat on the other side.

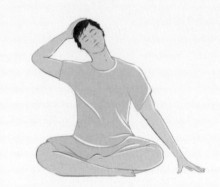

SEATED SIDE STRETCH

▸ From a seated position, gently inhale, lifting
  the left arm up towards the sky finding length
  in the side body. As you exhale take a side
  bend over to the right-hand side keeping the sit
  bones grounded.

▸ Inhale brings you up through centre then
  repeat on the other side.

▸ Repeat 5 times.

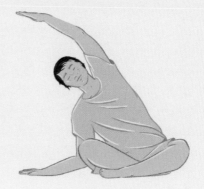

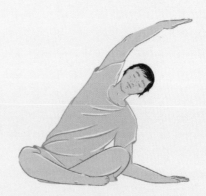

SEATED TWIST

▸ From a seated position, bring the right hand to the left knee and the left fingers tips behind you. Inhale to find length through the spine, growing tall through the crown of the head. As you exhale take a gentle twist gazing over your left shoulder. Imagine the twist going all the way up the spine (like a spiral staircase) avoiding just twisting the cervical spine (the neck).

▸ Hold this posture for 3-5 breaths and then slowly release before repeating on the opposite side.

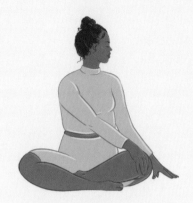

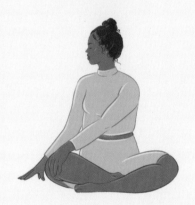

STANDING FORWARD FOLD POSE
(UTTANASANA)

▶ Stand at the top of the mat, feet hip distance apart, spine long and a small bend in the knees.

▶ Exhale and slowly hinge forward at the hips melting the torso towards the thighs, keeping the spine long.

▶ Bring the hands to the floor, to your shins or onto blocks placed on the mat in line with the shoulders (wherever is comfortable). Bend the knees as much as you need to keep length in the spine.

▶ Take 5 breaths here, then slowly return back to the upright position.

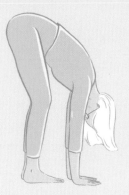

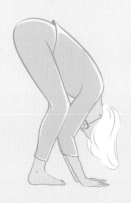

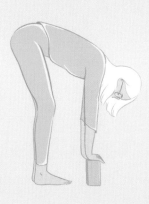

SUPINE TWIST

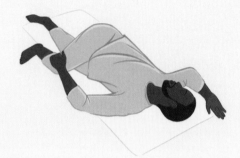

▶ Starting on your back, hug your right knee into your chest and gently start to rotate it over to the left-hand side, bringing your gaze to the right and stretching your right arm in line with your shoulder, or with a bend in the elbow.

▶ The left hand can come onto the knee to intensify the stretch. Try and keep the shoulders grounded, but if the knee doesn't touch the floor, that's okay. Hold for 5 breaths and repeat on the other side.

▶ Option to either extend the bent leg or bring both knees in and twist.

UPWARD-FACING DOG
(URDHVA MUKHA SVANASANA)

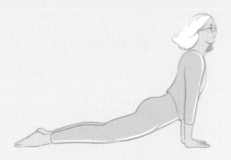

- Starting in plank pose (see page 167) slowly move the hips down and forwards squeezing the glutes and coming onto the tops of the feet, pressing them firmly into the floor.

- Keep the arms straight (take a gentle bend in the elbows to help open the chest), roll the shoulders back and down, opening through the heart space. Create a feeling of dragging the hands backwards and down into the mat to help draw the chest through the arms.

- Activate the front of your thighs, keep the knees lifted off the floor and hug the navel to spine. The glutes should be engaged to keep the pelvis neutral and avoid pinching the lower back.

- Gaze forwards and keep the neck long.

- Hold for 5 slow breaths and then slowly on an exhale hug navel to spine and slowly lift the hips up and back to downward-facing dog.

- Option to come into this pose from *chaturanga* (see page 180), coming onto the tops of the feet, straightening the arms and breathing the chest forward.

- If this doesn't feel like a good pose for your body, cobra pose (see page 158) can be a great modification.

WARRIOR II
(*VIRABHADRASANA II*)

- From downward-facing dog (see page 160), exhale and step the right foot between the hands (use your hand to help you if required).

- Inhale up to stand turning the hips open to the left side and coming onto the sole of the left foot. The outer edge of the left foot should be parallel to the back of the mat. The right foot is facing forward and the heel of the right foot is in line with the arch or heel of the left foot.

- Square the hips towards the side of the mat, keep the torso long, ribs drawing in, spine neutral and shoulders soft.

- Raise the arms so they are parallel to the floor and lengthen them in opposite directions. Gaze at the middle fingertip of the right hand.

- Exhale and bend into the right knee bringing it over the ankle, trying to bring the thigh as parallel to the floor as is comfortable. Press into the four corners of both feet to lift the arches and press the right inner knee outwards, engaging the glute so the knee doesn't collapse in.

- Take 5 breaths here then exhale as you windmill the hands back to the mat, framing the front foot before stepping back to downward-facing dog.

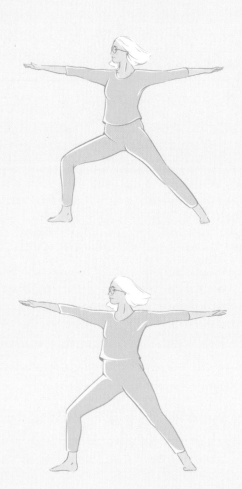

WARRIOR III
(*VIRABHADRASANA III*)

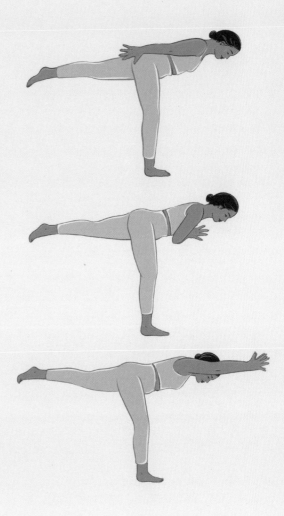

▸ From downward-facing dog (see page 160),
  exhale and step the right foot between the
  hands (use your hand to help you if required).

▸ Inhale up to standing, lifting the arms straight
  up to the ceiling. The hips are facing forward,
  right knee stacked over ankle. The left knee can
  have a slight bend to help keep the pelvis and
  spine neutral. This is high lunge.

▸ Exhale slowly shifting the weight forwards,
  hinging from the hips and bringing the left
  leg back up behind you, pointing the toes and
  squeezing the glutes. Push firmly through the
  grounded foot and big toe mound to activate
  the stabilising muscles in the hip. The left
  hip will want to lift up, try to square it in line
  with the right (placing the hands on the hips
  can be helpful).

▸ The spine stays long, creating a long line
  from the crown of your head to your left toes.
  The hands can come to the hips, heart centre,
  behind or reach out in front.

▸ Hold for 5 slow breaths.

▸ Inhale to return to high lunge, exhale back
  to downward-facing dog and repeat on the
  opposite side.

YOGA PUSH-UP
(*CHATURANGA*)

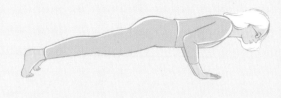

- ▶ Start in plank pose (see page 167) with the spine neutral, legs active, glutes on, core engaged and ribs drawing in.

- ▶ Exhale as you start to lower the body in one straight line, elbows pointing backwards. Have a sensation of 'dialing' the hands in opposite directions (like screwing jam jar lids) and pulling back with the hands to keep the shoulder tips lifted (the hands don't actually move). Lower as much as you can control or until the upper arms make a 90-degree angle with the floor; avoid the head and shoulders dipping down.

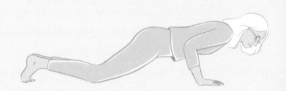

- ▶ Hold for 1–5 breaths. Either inhale and lift into upward-facing dog (see page 177), or exhale and push back up to plank.

- ▶ Option to lower the intensity by dropping the knees, this is a challenging posture so tune in and be mindful of your body.

FURTHER READING

The books and article listed here delve deeper into some of the subjects covered in *Yoga Happy*. Whether you want more information on the *yamas* and *niyamas*, the *chakras*, *pranayama*, or simply ways to further your self-practice, these resources are a great place to start.

Ashtanga Yoga: The Practice Manual, David Swenson

Breath, James Nestor

Eastern Body Western Mind, Anodea Judith

Embrace Yoga's Roots, Susanna Barkati

Frontiers in Psychology: Forever Young(er): potential age-defying effects of long-term meditation on gray matter atrophy, Eileen Luders, Nicola Cherbuin, Florian Kurth

How Yoga Works, Geshe Michael Roach

Light on Yoga, B. K. S. Iyengar

Teaching Yoga Beyond the Poses, Sage Rountree and Alexandra Desiato

The Bhagavad Gita, Veda Viyasa

The Book of Yoga Self-Practice, Rebecca Anderton-Davies

The Effortless Mind, Will Williams

The Four Agreements, Don Miguel Ruiz

The Hatha Yoga Pradipika, Swami Muktibodhananda

The Mind Illuminated, Culadasa (John Yates PhD) and Matthew Immergut PhD with Jeremy Graves

The Miracle of Mindfulness, Thich Nhat Hanh

The Tree of Yoga, B. K. S. Iyengar

The Untethered Soul, Michael Singer

The Yamas and Niyamas, Deborah Adele

The Yoga Sutras, Nicolai Bachman

The Yoga Sutras of Patañjali, translation and commentary by Sri Swami Satchidananda

What Is Mindfulness, Dr Tamara Russell

Yoga Anatomy, Kaminoff Matthews

INDEX

Note: page numbers in **bold** refer to diagrams.

ABOUT THE AUTHOR

Hannah Barrett is an international yoga teacher who empowers students all over the world to feel confident and find strength on the mat.

After the traumatic birth of her daughter, yoga helped Hannah rediscover who she was and find her purpose in life. The transformational effect and growth yoga had on Hannah's recovery gave her passion to help others find strength and calm in the chaos of their life through yoga.

Hannah has undertaken 200 hours Ashtanga Vinyasa training with Yoga London and 300 hours LYT Comprehensive Anatomy training. She also has a further 150 hours covering prenatal, postnatal and mandala training.

Hannah is known for her strength-based creative flows and a style that is playful, anatomy-based and challenging but always accessible. Her intention is always to empower you to create strength, resilience and connection, feel grounded and have fun in the process.

Website: www.hannahbarrettyoga.com
Instagram: @hannahbarrettyoga

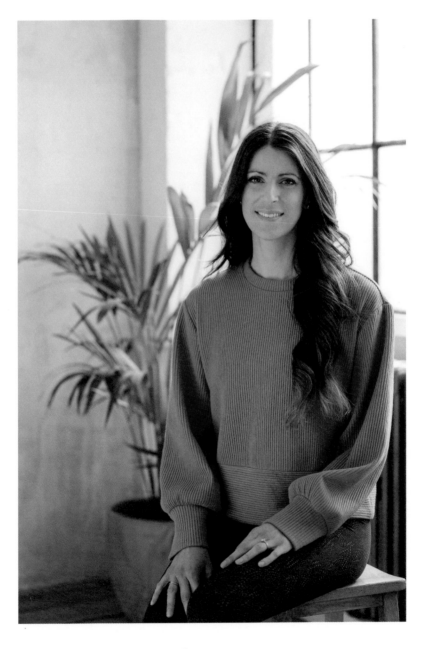

ACKNOWLEDGEMENTS

I am grateful to so many people for making *Yoga Happy* come to life.

A huge thank you to my literary agent Jenny Heller who helped me craft *Yoga Happy* from the beginning and made sure we ended up with a team whose vision matched ours. You were, and continue to be, my sounding board and I am so happy to have you in my life.

Thank you to the whole team at Quadrille, in particular Sarah Lavelle and Gemma Hayden who truly turned my dream into a reality and were an absolute pleasure to work alongside.

And to my wonderful editor Imogen Fortes. You are incredibly patient, insightful and hard-working and I couldn't have asked for a better editor. Thank you for believing in *Yoga Happy* and in me.

To illustrator Eleanor Hardiman who really did bring everything I envisioned to life in the most incredible way. To my lovely friend Cecilia Cristolovean – I could not have imagined anyone else doing the photography. You are a pure talent and I am grateful to have had you as part of *Yoga Happy*.

Thank you to my teachers and students, for everything you have taught and continue to teach me, and for inspiring me every single day to do my best. I appreciate you more than you know. If you are holding this book in your hands, thank you for allowing me and my yoga passion into your life. I hope it changes your life as much as it has mine.

Thank you to my wonderful family: Mum, Dad and Oliver – I love you. Thank you for always loving and supporting me.

Thank you to my in-laws, the Barrett clan, who are awesome and make life more fun. And to the Belgian crew, whom I don't see enough, but whenever I do I have the best time.

This book was created during lockdown –thank you to all my friends who made pandemic life bearable. I am forever grateful and value you so much.

Giles, you have always believed in and supported me and it was you that gave me that first push to follow my yoga dream. I love you. Thank you also for creating a beautiful writing studio for me, even if it did get flooded a week later, never to be used again.

And to my babies Jack and Amelie. Thank for teaching me so much about the joy of childhood and motherhood and how to be truly present. Thank you for making my life better and showing me love I could never have imagined.

PUBLISHING DIRECTOR Sarah Lavelle
EDITOR Imogen Fortes
SENIOR DESIGNER Gemma Hayden
PHOTOGRAPHER Cecilia Cristolovean
ILLUSTRATOR Eleanor Hardiman
HEAD OF PRODUCTION Stephen Lang
PRODUCTION CONTROLLER Katie Jarvis

Published in 2022 by Quadrille,
an imprint of Hardie Grant Publishing

Quadrille
52–54 Southwark Street
London SE1 1UN
quadrille.com

Cataloguing in Publication Data: a catalogue record
for this book is available from the British Library.

ISBN 978 1 78713 767 7
Printed in China

This book is not intended as a substitute for genuine
medical advice. The reader should consult a medical
professional in matters relating to their health.

The publisher would like to thank Varley
(uk.varley.com) and Liforme (liforme.com)
for the generous loan of clothing and mats
for the photoshoot.

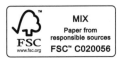

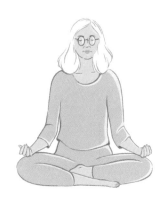